THE BURFORD NDU MODEL

Caring in Practice

Edited by

CHRISTOPHER JOHNS

RGN, RMN, Cert.Ed, MN
Reader in Advanced Nursing Practice
University of Luton

**Blackwell
Science**

> *To practitioners everywhere, who continuously strive*
> *to make their visions of nursing a caring reality.*

© 1994 by Blackwell Science Ltd
Editorial Offices:
Osney Mead, Oxford OX2 0EL
25 John Street, London WC1N 2BL
23 Ainslie Place, Edinburgh EH3 6AJ
238 Main Street, Cambridge,
  Massachusetts 02142, USA
54 University Street, Carlton,
  Victoria 3053, Australia

Other Editorial Offices:
Arnette Blackwell SA
1, rue de Lille
75007 Paris
France

Blackwell Wissenschafts-Verlag GmbH
Kurfürstendamm 57
10707 Berlin
Germany

Blackwell MZV
Feldgasse 13
1238 Wien
Austria

First published 1994

Set by DP Photosetting, Aylesbury, Bucks
Printed and bound in Great Britain by
Hartnolls Ltd., Bodmin, Cornwall.

DISTRIBUTORS

Marston Book Services Ltd
PO Box 87
Oxford OX2 0DT
(*Orders:* Tel: 0865 791155
        Fax: 0865 791927
        Telex: 837515)

USA
Blackwell Science, Inc.
238 Main Street
Cambridge, MA 02142
(*Orders:* Tel: 800 759-6102
        617 876-7000)

Canada
Times Mirror Professional Publishing Ltd
130 Flaska Drive
Markham, Ontario L6G 1B8
(*Orders:* Tel: 800 268-4178
        416 470-6739)

Australia
Blackwell Science Pty Ltd
54 University Street
Carlton, Victoria 3053
(*Orders:* Tel: (03) 347-5552)

British Library
Cataloguing in Publication Data

A catalogue record for this book is available
from the British Library

ISBN 0–632–03886–1

Library of Congress
Cataloging in Publication Data

The Burford NDU model : caring in practice/
  edited by Christopher Johns.
      p. cm.
  Includes bibliographical references and
index.
  ISBN 0-632-03886-1
  1. Nursing–Philosophy. 2. Nursing–
England–Burford (Oxfordshire)
3. Nursing models. I. Johns, Christopher.
  [DNLM: 1. Philosophy, Nursing.
2. Models, Nursing. 3. Holistic Health.
WY 86 B953 1994]
RT84.5.B87 1994
610.73′01—dc 20
DNLM/DLC
for Library of Congress   94-12532
                                      CIP

Contents

List of Contributors

SUSAN BOOKER RGN, ONC, Primary nurse/Team leader, Oxford Community Hospital.
Has used the BNDU model in her work.

KATE BUTCHER BA(Hons), RGN, Associate nurse, 7e NDU, Oxford Radcliffe Hospital.
Commenced work at Burford in September 1991. Burford was her first post after qualifying at Sheffield Polytechnic with a degree in nursing.

ROGER COWELL BA, SEN(G), RGN, Primary nurse, Burford Community Hospital.
Commenced work at Burford in September 1991.

JAN DEWING RGN, DN (London), Dip.N.Ed, MN, BA, Head of the Burford NDU, Lecturer/Practitioner at Oxford Brookes University, Manager of Burford Community Hospital.
Commenced work at Burford in April 1992.

ROBERT GARBETT RGN, BN(Hons), Project worker/Team leader, 7e NDU, Oxford Radcliffe Hospital.
Has used the BNDU model in his work.

CHRISTOPHER JOHNS RGN, RMN, Cert.Ed, MN, Reader in Advanced Nursing Practice, University of Luton.
Head of the Burford NDU between January 1989 and December 1991. Elected to Epsilon beta chapter, Sigma Theta Tau in 1994.

CAROL McCAFFREY
Currently a fourth-year student on the undergraduate nursing programme in the School of Health Care Studies, Oxford Brookes University.

BRENDAN McCORMACK BSc(Hons) Nursing, DPSN, PGCEA, RGN, RMN, Development and Research Fellow/Clinical Lecturer in Nursing, a three-way appointment between the National Institute for Nursing, Oxford, School of Health Care Studies, Oxford Brookes University and Oxford Community Health NHS Trust based at Oxford Community Hospital.

Worked closely with Christopher Johns, primary nurses and other staff during October 1991 in order to extend the Burford model into other care settings.

SUSAN METCALF SRN, SCM, NDU Cert, CPT, District nurse and clinical practice teacher.

Has used the BNDU model in her work.

BART O'BRIEN RGN, Dip.App.Sci (Nsg), BNsg, PhD, Assistant Director of Nursing – Clinical, Julia Farr Centre, Adelaide, South Australia.

Has been working to establish two NDUs at Julia Farr Centre since 1991.

JUDITH POPE RGN, RM, Dip.App.Sci (Nsg), Clinical Nurse Consultant, H6A NDU, Julia Farr Centre, Adelaide, South Australia.

Has been working to develop the ward as an NDU since 1991, taking a leadership/mentorship role.

LYN SUTHERLAND RGN, ITU Cert, Dip.HE(DN), District nurse, Jericho Health Centre, Oxford.

Worked at Burford as a primary nurse between September 1990 and September 1991. She had previously been a sister of an acute oncology unit.

Foreword

In the current 'modern' health care climate, there is increasing agreement that nursing education and health care are in a state of disequilibrium and that the institutional, scientific and technological orientation of today's health and nursing care systems cannot be sustained into the 21st century. Without attention to a paradigm of health and human caring that integrates nursing's philosophy and values with its functional care activities, the inevitable conclusion is that education and practice derived from, and perpetuating, outdated functional 'doing' orientations will result in nurses ill-equipped to meet the challenges they face during a post-modern era.

International studies and commissions, reports and research around the world indicate a growing consensus between and among the public and the nursing, medical and health community regarding health care reform measures and the need for parallel educational and practice reform at all levels. There is open agreement worldwide that the modern health care industry is really a sick treatment care system – a system that was built upon an industrial model which differentiated technical from professional work, and which separated education and practice from scholarship and research. Such a model is deemed increasingly archaic and dysfunctional. In its place are emerging professional education and practice models requiring more multi-disciplinary, broad-based, integrated caring–healing practice values, knowledge and skills; models that attend to praxis activities that seek to both integrate and transform the nurse's personal and professional values, beliefs and reflective acts with clinical decision-making in the concrete world of practice.

As this work points out, 'all models of nursing are implicitly and explicitly underwritten by the assumptions of their authors concerning the nature of nursing'. It can likewise be acknowledged that all nursing practice is implicitly and explicitly influenced by the practising nurses' views and values concerning the nature of nursing. However, one of the breakdowns in contemporary nursing practice is the separation of reflection from action; a tendency toward acts, but not toward asking; a tendency to leap in without becoming conscious or reflective about leaping back or leaping ahead; a proclivity to disconnect one's theory or views about the nature of nursing from one's practice of nursing; a reluctance to integrate one's philosophy with one's action.

Finally, 'modern' nursing has an affinity, almost a bias, toward carrying out functional, concrete skills, that satisfy the technical accountability demands of a medical treatment regime or an institutional bureaucratic demand, before making itself directly accountable to the public for its caring, healing, health knowledge and practices that are informed by its values, philosophy, knowledge and skills. The profession in both education and practice has tended to yield to the bureaucratic–institutional technical culture demands, rather than developing and emerging in its own, more completely actualized professional health and human caring model.

In nursing education and research, there has been the past history of attempts by modern science to mimic a medical science model which limited nursing science to restrictive thinking related to empirical knowledge as the primary way of knowing, while rejecting at worst, or at best not honoring, nursing's diverse and whole ways of knowing and being. Such limited emphasis of empirical and behaviourist science eclipsed caring from being foundational to nursing knowledge and practice; eclipsed and silenced nursing's values and philosophy, and caring ethos from its natural prominence and place in the health care system. Moreover, such distortions during the rise of 'modern' technical medicine were compounded by the culture of a patriarchal system further restricting nursing from its full development as a distinct discipline within both practice and academic settings.

However, during the past two-to-three decades, nursing scholars and clinicians at multiple levels have been questioning and revising nursing's very foundations for education, practice and research. Such efforts have resulted in the critique of the dominant ideology of the patriarchal system; have led to the generation of multiple nursing theories, clinical nursing research and theory-based practice models; have led to a revisiting of nursing ethics, basic philosophical beliefs and ultimately to a re-examining of what is intended and needed for truly professional nursing practice.

During the 1980s, further important discourses emerged across developed countries about the nature of nursing science. These discourses critiqued nursing's 'modern' epistemological emphasis on empiricism, and critiqued the lack of ontological–philosophical–moral–ethical clarity about the nature of 'being'; about the nature of person, caring, health, illness and environment; and about the nature of nursing itself. This discourse has brought new voice to nursing's place in health care; has now led to new perspectives about the nature of nursing's paradigm and the role of caring values and knowledge in theory and in practice.

Part of nursing's self-critique and revision of the profession is related to nursing coming of age, growing up as both a discipline and profession; is related to nursing gaining philosophical, moral, ontological, epistemological and pragmatic clarity about its subject matter and its phenomena of interest, in both theory and practice.

Such critique, reflection and study of foundational issues about nursing are related to the fact that nursing is becoming increasingly critical about its practice. This 'becoming critical' is related to a recommitment to values and perspectives about human caring, about human–environment–caring therapeutic connections and nursing-sensitive patient outcomes; is related to how basic foundational beliefs about such concepts, directly or indirectly, influence one's very acts, one's instrumental and expressive, moral and pragmatic actions in practice.

Finally this revision of nursing is related to a reconnecting, a re-membering of its values, traditions and beliefs during a modern century dominated by technology, cure and economic–bureaucratic metaphors which have distorted and silenced nursing's values and practice.

However, nursing's re-connection with its roots and basic values is now, at the professional practice level, beginning to have an impact on the health and healing of individuals, families and communities. At the disciplinary level, this re-connection and re-vision is allowing for a more actualized health and human caring profession to emerge for a new century, in the best tradition of Florence Nightingale. Such maturity positions nursing to truly come of age and awaken to its power to publicly and scholastically address the health challenges of these post-modern times.

This book about the Burford Nursing Development Unit provides a model of scholarly therapeutic practice, contributing to the further development of both the discipline and profession of nursing through a return to its philosophical basis for reflective caring practice and knowledge generation. Further, this work helps to explicate the details of a professional practice model that can serve as a guide and paradigm case for transforming clinical nursing care as nursing seeks to respond to the public's cry for health care reform now and into the future.

Finally, as the year 2000 approaches us, this work is a living reminder and beacon for others who wish to challenge the critics who say that philosophy and theory are not relevant to changing nursing practice for a new era. The Burford Community Hospital Nursing Development model, as described in this book, not only reminds us of nursing's potential as a profession, but also reminds us of our social mandate to improve our practice and come of age as a full health and human caring profession, better serving the public now and into the 21st century.

Dr Jean Watson PhD, RN, FAAN
Distinguished Professor of Nursing
Director of the Center for Human Caring
University of Colorado Health Sciences Center
Denver, Colorado, USA

Preface

Burford Community Hospital is a small community hospital nestled in the rural Cotswold hills of Oxfordshire. It became well-known as a centre of creative practice from 1983 through the work of Alan Pearson, and asserted itself as a nursing development unit in 1983. Since that time it has endeavoured to contribute to the development of nursing knowledge. Indeed, to do less it would fail in its own defined sense of the purpose of a nursing development unit – to be creative in practice, to appropriately evaluate this creative practice, and to share this work with the world in appropriate forms.

In 1989, shortly after my appointment as hospital manager and clinical leader, I commenced a process of reflection on the nature and purpose of nursing at Burford and how this was interpreted in practice. The foundation for this work was to articulate a clear vision of what nursing was at Burford and to explore ways in which this vision could become a reality in everyday practice. In doing so, it explicitly built on previous developments in nursing practice pioneered by Alan Pearson.

As a result, four discrete but interrelated ways of implementing the vision or philosophy for practice were developed and carried out (see figure below).

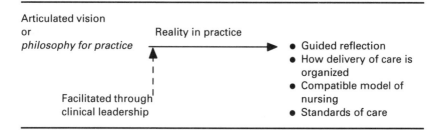

Ways of implementing a philosophy.

The interrelationship of the Burford Nursing Development Unit model with standards of care and guided reflection will become apparent in the first two chapters within the unifying thread of reflective practice.

This book explicates the development of a compatible model for nursing practice – the Burford Nursing Development Unit Holistic Model for Nursing Practice, or simply the BNDU model. The structure of this model has previously been published (Johns 1991) and narratives of the model in use have been published as case studies (Johns 1990; Sutherland 1991). All names used in the case studies are fictitious.

This model is offered for use by practitioners in any nursing context, not as a prescription of how practice should be, but as a reflexive tool and heuristic device that enables practitioners to realize their beliefs about their practice.

I realize that readers may be tempted to reify the model and interpret it as prescription, but let me try to persuade you not to do that. If you feel that the beliefs and values you identify as meaningful for you in your practice are similar to those espoused within Burford's philosophy for practice, then you may only need to adapt the model slightly to reflect your own practice. If on the other hand your beliefs are quite different, then you can take the principles that underpin the BNDU model to build your own along similar pathways. That you have beliefs and values about the nature of your practice is without question, although gaining access to these and expressing them in a meaningful way is not necessarily easy to achieve.

I am indebted to Jean Watson, for her contribution to writing the foreword to this book and for her work in expanding nurses' horizons of nursing as human caring. Jean sets out the context and agenda for a nursing paradigm based on human caring and human science. The clear message is that nursing needs to emerge from the shadows of medical domination to fulfil its caring role in responding to and meeting the health needs of communities.

The John Radcliffe Hospital, Oxford is now known as the newly created trust, the Oxford Radcliffe Hospital. I have used the new name throughout this book.

Chapters 1 and 2 set out the key issues in the model's development. In doing so I expand on earlier, more tentative work (Johns 1991). The following seven chapters represent how practitioners at Burford and elsewhere have used the BNDU model in their practice. Chapters 3, 4 and 5 are reflective accounts by Burford practitioners who work or have worked at Burford. Chapters 6, 7, 8 and 9 are written by practitioners who have applied or have been influenced by the BNDU model in the context of their own practice. In each case these contributors/practitioners were asked to write a personal and reflective account that:

(1) critiqued their use of the model
(2) where possible described the use of the model with case study.

The results are very personal accounts or narratives of engagement with the BNDU model which itself reflects how nursing practice and knowledge becomes personal and creative when nurses are given the opportunity or are able to create the opportunity to make it so.

As a consequence these accounts are different. I have written an editor's commentary for each contribution, included at the end of each chapter, to highlight some key issues that have been explicated in theory in the first two chapters. The concluding chapter offers my personal viewpoint as an 'insider'.

Christopher Johns (Editor)

References

Johns, C.C. (1990) Double Dilemma. *Nursing Times*, **86**(50), 47–9.
Johns, C.C. (1991) The Burford Nursing Development Unit holistic model of nursing practice. *Journal of Advanced Nursing*, **16**, 1090–98.
Sutherland, L. (1991) The Burford Model. *Nursing*, **4**(25), 19–21.

Acknowledgements

The quotations from Sacks (1991) *Awakenings* and Forster (1989) *Have the men had enough?* are reproduced with permission. I also wish to thank Lynne Batehup for her critical reading and insights; Jean Watson for her contribution and inspiration; Alan Pearson for his vision; and the staff of Blackwell Science Ltd, especially Lisa Field and Teresa Heapy for their encouragement and Julie Musk for her editing.

Robert Garbett wishes to acknowledge Mary FitzGerald, former lecturer practitioner on 7e NDU without whom none of the work described in Chapter 7 would have taken place. He also wishes to thank Nigel Northcott for his support and helpful comments.

Part I
Philosophy

Chapter 1
A Philosophical Basis for Nursing Practice

Christopher Johns

'Theory without practice is vacuous, but practice without theory is like someone going to sea without a map in a ship without a rudder [Clark 1982 cited by Jackson 1986] ... it is important too, that the map you choose gets you where you want to go, and the ship you sail in doesn't sink before you get there.' (Jackson 1986, p.26)

Choosing a model of nursing for practice

Without doubt using a model of nursing is *de rigueur* for those practitioners with any pretension for developing their clinical practice. Yet, is the use of a model of nursing merely a conceptually attractive artefact or is it something which can really facilitate practitioners to practise more creatively and more effectively?

All models of nursing are explicitly and implicitly underwritten by the assumptions that their authors hold concerning the nature of nursing. As such, there can only be two ways that practitioners can sensibly utilize a model of nursing as a framework for their practice – either by matching their own assumptions about the nature of nursing against the assumptions that underpin the various available models of nursing, and then to choose the most compatible, or to use their own assumptions to construct a 'tailor-made' model of nursing.

This position rejects any eclectic approach that puts together bits of different models to construct a 'hybrid' model. This rejection is because models of nursing aim to portray a complete realization of nursing practice and in this sense have integrity. Pulling different models apart and creating a hybrid model must inevitably destroy the internal coherence and integrity of the models used. The counter argument is that practitioners who choose to construct such a model must themselves address the issues of internal coherence and integrity.

Beliefs and values

However, it may not be easy for practitioners to be sensible. Without doubt, nurses have struggled to relate to the assumptions that underpin the various models of nursing. The language of models and the implicit nature of many of the models' assumptions have not helped this process. As Miller (1985, p. 423) remarked in exploring the relationship between nursing theory and nursing practice:

> 'Many nursing theories and models are so abstract and so complex that it is virtually impossible to see their relevance to practice.'

Miller suggests that nurses will have difficulty getting access to the models' assumptions upon which to make a meaningful decision as to which model to choose.

Such access, of course, depends on the practitioners' articulation of their own assumptions (I prefer to say their beliefs and values) about the nature of their nursing practice, in order to match them. In fact both these 'sensible' methods of utilizing a model of nursing require that practitioners have articulated their own beliefs and values.

This may be difficult to achieve because nurses, at least in the UK, have generally had a functional orientation to nursing practice. In this sense, nurses have tended to view nursing in terms of what they do rather than as a reflection of their beliefs and values about what nursing is. I believe that this functional orientation reflects how nurses have tended to choose a model based on its functional use, and, in particular, its assessment strategy. This emphasis on function is probably the major reason why nurses struggle to write and implement coherent philosophies of care (or of practice – Johns 1991) because they do not conceptualize nursing in a philosophic mode. As a consequence, this is probably why the Roper, Logan and Tierney Activities of Living Model (1980) is so popular in this country, because it most reflects what nurses already do.

As one commentator on nursing models put it:

> 'The advantage of models based on activities of living is that they are easy to understand and fit in with the personal value systems of many nurses.' (Luker 1988, p.28)

This functional orientation predicts that nursing models will have a minimal impact on the way nursing is practised. The chosen model will be merely overlaid on what practitioners already do rather than profoundly change practice. As Luker concludes her paper (p.29):

'Formal models of nursing may be a passing craze which community nurses can well afford to miss out on. In some sense formal models offer little more than an illusion that change for the better is on the way and it is in this sense that formal models are red herrings.'

Luker reflects a belief that external factors such as formal models are instrumental to change and suggests their impact will be minimal. Of course, she is absolutely right. Forces for change around philosophical or theoretical concepts are unlikely to flourish in a culture of 'nursing as doing' unless it has some obvious utility value.

The proof of this statement lies like debris around the chaos wreaked in the name of the nursing process. The nursing process had immediate functional appeal and yet it has always struggled to flourish and to influence practice. Its explicit philosophical message around the concept of individualized care has been largely obscured. In comparison, what hope do nursing models have beyond a functional interpretation and the immediacy offered by check list type assessment strategies?

A broad consequence of a functional approach to choosing a model of nursing as a framework for guiding practice is that the model's underlying philosophical assumptions are either disregarded or accepted uncritically. As an 'offered' framework for framing reality, a model intends to be prescriptive or instrumental.

This 'instrumental' intention of models of nursing is reflected in the work of Aggleton and Chalmers (1987). They claim that strong models are predictive of outcomes whilst specifying the beliefs and values they should have and the interventions nurses should use. They also outline the criteria against which a conceptual model can be evaluated. The risk of such a normative approach to nursing practice reduces the role of the nurse to that of a technician applying a certain set of rules. Such an approach has certain consequences. As Webb (1986a, p.7) enlightens us:

'This mechanistic view of human-beings denies their very humanity and treats them like computers which receive input, process it automatically and without thinking, and produce output.'

If models of nursing are to be useful to practitioners then clearly they need to influence how practitioners practise. Intuitively nurse practitioners know that such an approach stifles their own humanity and that of their patients.

An alternative to the 'instrumental' approach to model building is the 'reflective' approach as advocated by the BNDU model. This approach intends to reflect how practitioners actually think and feel about their nursing.

Models of nursing portray visions of how nursing can be (Meleis 1985). The instrumental approach specifies this vision as ideology. An ideology is a belief system and has attendant attitudes held as true and valid which shape a group's interpretation of reality and behaviour and are used to justify and legitimate actions (Mezirow 1981). The discerning practitioner sifting through the plethora of nursing models may well ask, 'Why are there so many and disparate views of nursing?'

Commentators such as Fawcett (1984) have attempted to establish a meta-paradigm of nursing based on common elements within all models, that is, how the practitioner perceives nursing, client, health and environment, and the impression drawn from the literature on nursing models is that this has become a widely accepted or normative view against which models are judged as valid.

This is not to say that what practitioners actually feel and think about their nursing is not influenced by ideology. Such a notion is clearly absurd, for, as I shall describe later in this chapter, the concepts within the BNDU model are strongly influenced by ideology. However, the significant difference between an instrumental approach and a reflective approach is that what practitioners feel and think about their nursing is always being challenged through reflection on their practice. In this way, an ideology becomes personalized and hence meaningful for practitioners.

Of course there will always be a gap between practitioners' visions of nursing and the way nursing is practised. As Rawnsley (1990, p.42) so eloquently puts it:

'Caring may be a desirable image for nursing, but is it meaningful? Is there congruence between the lived experience of nursing practice and the intellectual pursuit of caring as nursing's professional crest? When living the reality of their practice, nurses need ways through which they can connect the conceptual concerns of the discipline with the raw data of experience.'

In this sense, nursing models reflect the dialectic between ideology and experience.

model of nursing

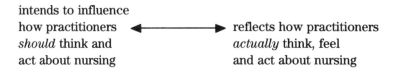

intends to influence
how practitioners   ◄━━━━━━━►   reflects how practitioners
should think and   *actually* think, feel
act about nursing   and act about nursing

Neither dialectic is static; each is continually changing in the light of reflection. As such, a reflective nursing model, as a blueprint for practice, must itself be responsive to account for this shifting tension between ideology and experience.

Connecting

There are different ways that practitioners can connect the raw data of their experiences with the conceptual concerns of the discipline, assuming that these conceptual concerns are reflected in a statement of the practitioners' shared beliefs and values.

This book is primarily concerned with how choosing a compatible model of nursing to act as a framework of practice can make this connection. Other ways of connecting are:

(1) the method practitioners choose to organize the delivery of care to patients
(2) through setting standards of care
(3) through reflective practice.

These methods do not exist in isolation from each other. Rather, a critical approach to nursing will utilize each of these means. Whilst I have recognized these concepts as discrete, the interconnection between each of them will become more apparent as I unfold the BNDU model of nursing.

Besides the choice of organizational method to deliver the care to the patient, the key underlying concept within setting standards of care and reflective practice and a compatible model for nursing practice is reflection.

Reflection

Reflective practice involves the practitioner paying attention to 'significant' aspects of experience in order to make sense of it within the context of their intention. By reflecting on and taking action to resolve the contradictions between espoused beliefs and actual practice within each experience, practitioners come to know themselves within the context of their work and learns to become increasingly effective in achieving desired work.

In setting standards of care, practitioners reflect on a discrete aspect of practice, such as how pain is managed, or the privacy offered to patients, or the comfort of patients. This reflection is focused on care processes and outcomes with particular patients.

Presumably practitioners who intend to choose a model of nursing 'off the shelf' will need to pay attention to a number of 'reflective' questions before they can sensibly choose the most compatible model to suit their practice:

- What are the assumptions that support this particular model?
- What sense can we make of the particular concepts within the model?
- Are the assumptions within the model valid as a foundation for our own practice?
- Do these assumptions match with our own beliefs about the nature of our practice?
- Does the model work in practice?
- How does this model help us achieve what we are trying to achieve?
- How do we interpret this model for our practice?
- What sort of development do we need before we can practically implement this model?

In other words, within a reflective approach, it is not or necessarily should not be easy to choose a model 'off the shelf'. Hence, how much more difficult for practitioners to sensibly choose bits from several models unless the bits are chosen for their functional attraction?

The reflective approach is implicitly critical, in contrast with the instrumental approach that encourages nurses to adopt a non-critical stance and that denies practitioners the need to articulate their own beliefs and values about nursing and in the process seduces practitioners into a web of conceptual attraction and illusion which ultimately lacks meaning.

Benner and Wrubel (1989, p.83) note that:

'When the person/situation are analysed into objective lists, meaningful distinctions are lost and it is hard to determine which aspects of the situation are most important.'

Many nurses are now articulating their beliefs and values in written statements or 'philosophies of care' which create the potential for a more critical approach to the use of nursing models in practice, whether 'off the shelf' or by constructing models such as the BNDU model as described within this book.

Developing a model from the beliefs and values of the practitioners who work together assumes that practice is not driven by or detached from theory, but asserts that it is informed, critical, reflexive and committed. In other words, practice has become 'praxis' (Carr & Kemmis 1986, p.33). Within this belief, the theory–practice 'gap' becomes merely a contradiction between 'what should be done' and 'what is actually practised', and a natural focus for the reflective practitioner to take appropriate action to resolve these contradictions towards achieving effective and congruent work.

Meleis (1985, p.301) highlights the importance of nursing models in moving the boundaries of nursing forward. In doing so she also highlights the ideal nature of nursing models. She states:

> 'Existing nursing theories tended to address imaginative and ideal nursing practice that did not really exist except in the minds of their creators. Theirs were visions of what nursing ought to be and what care should be like; theirs were necessary visions of how nursing should move forward to establish its identity and its boundaries. Now that we have ideal goals, modifications of these theories will ensue as nurses begin to describe and document what is there and what goals are attainable.'

Meleis's claim that nursing theories in the form of nursing models, or for that matter in any form, have moved forward the boundaries of practice is problematic. I have a deep uneasiness about nursing if it requires nursing models to tell human-beings (nurses) that other human-beings (patients and their families) are in reality also human-beings. This is a deeply shocking notion that reflects how reductionist nursing practice and health care in general has become. Human-beings are clearly not objects to be taken apart. Meleis suggests that nursing models can now be modified 'as nurses begin to describe and document what is there and what is attainable.'

If I interpret Meleis correctly, she advocates a revisionist position which I feel is limited because it does not take into account the reality of where most nurses are coming from. It is as if there are two worlds: on one hand there is the world of theory – based on a theoretical account of practice; on the other hand there is the world of practice – based on a functional and largely uncritical and unarticulated account of what nurses actually do. Meleis suggests that these worlds can be easily linked.

This revisionist position is weak because the prescriptive approach of nursing models by its very nature precludes nurses, already entrenched in the functional perspective of nursing, from having to think critically about what it is they do. In deciding to use a model of nursing to guide practice, practitioners can only start from where they are. There are no short cuts or conceptual leaps to be achieved.

In many situations practitioners may consider they have not been involved in deciding which model to use. This may be prescribed as hospital or educational policy or by an individual in the exercise of his or her clinical authority. In such cases the model becomes prescribed. Change theory predicts that such prescription will result in lack of meaning for practitioners who are expected to use the model in practice. Ottaway (1976) has identified that for change to be meaningful, those affected by the change need to feel involved and have a sense of ownership. This is because change is deeply threatening. Failure to do this, inevitably leads to resistance and mere compliance rather than meaningful change.

However, such change clearly needs leadership. It needs someone who can enable practitioners to explore the issues and facilitate meaning. Hence, the change leaders need to 'contract' with practitioners they work with (Ottaway 1976).

This may be difficult unless the change leader enables the practitioners to feel 'free' to participate in such contracting. This may be a particular problem in traditional nursing organizations based on rigid hierarchical patterns where practitioners may feel powerless to participate. Where practitioners have clear responsibility for managing a caseload, for example with primary nurses, then hierarchical management patterns become contradictory. However, this is not to say that hierarchical patterns do not persist even in units that have implemented primary nursing. Nurses socialized into hierarchical ways of relating to others may find this difficult to unlearn and develop 'collegial' ways of working as outlined by Beyer and Marshall (1981).

The essence of collegiality is mutual ways of working with each other which can be considered necessary for practitioners to feel a sense of ownership. This sense of ownership is clearly reinforced with the implementation of primary nursing. In this system the traditional role of the ward sister of delegating work to staff to carry out and maintaining a supervisory role to ensure the work is being done competently, becomes redundant.

However, this is not without potential problems. In devolving the management of patient care to individual nurses it is reasonable to assume that primary nurses have a right to decide which model of nursing they wish to utilize in their practice – given the assumption that the major purpose of any model of nursing must be to offer the practitioner an appropriate framework from which they can coherently plan, give and communicate their nursing praxis. However, such a scenario would surely lead to chaos with the potential plethora of numerous models of nursing being used in one practice. Hence I am going to assume that it is preferable to have only one model of nursing. I believe this is a reasonable assumption to make with the emergence of a collective and agreed philosophy for practice.

Primary nurses, like all nurses, midwives and health visitors are not independent practitioners; in theory at least, it must be assumed that they work collectively towards defined outcomes in mutually compatible ways. As such, they need systems that reflect this essential collective nature of their work.

The decision to sensibly use a model of nursing in practice must therefore commence at the point where practitioners are. This point recognizes that change is both a social and historical process. Burford had chosen to use the Roper, Logan and Tierney model (1980) in 1983 (Pearson 1983). Pearson felt (p.53) that this model gave a 'global concept of nursing' and 'pointed out the knowledge base needed by all nurses and identified the uniqueness of nursing.' It is pertinent to note that Pearson also felt (p.53) that the model:

'... speaks to nurses in a language which is familiar and related to nursing in this country and hence its greatest advantage then is its ability to convey meaning to clinical nurses.'

These quotes suggest that Pearson chose a model of nursing that most fitted what nurses already do, supporting my earlier argument about a functional and prescriptive approach.

Pearson had also introduced the philosophy of care from the Loeb Center (Hall 1964) as the philosophical basis for practice at Burford and more generally as a philosophy for nursing as a distinct therapy separate from medicine. With hindsight, the significant weakness of this approach was the failure to integrate the Loeb philosophy with the decision to use the Roper *et al.* model. It was as if these two things stood alone.

The disadvantage of 'importing' a ready-made philosophy for practice is that it discourages practitioners from exploring and articulating their own practice. This is of course a similar argument to choosing a model of nursing 'off the shelf'. For model assumptions read the theorist's philosophy of care.

Pearson (1983, p.55) recognizes the evolutionary nature of his approach:

'No model can be accepted as final representation of reality, but only as a basis for further analysis, concept identification and theory building and testing leading to a dynamic and developing approach to the practice of nursing.'

At that time the use of Roper *et al.*'s model of nursing at Burford was clearly articulated and justified through Pearson's writings (1983; 1988).

Reflection on the continued use of the Roper, Logan and Tierney model of nursing at Burford

In October 1988 I brought together primary and district nurses at Burford to reflect on the continued use of the Roper *et al.* model of nursing in light of the hospital's newly developed philosophy for practice. The district nurses had not been part of the development of the philosophy yet it was useful to involve them because of their experience of using the Roper *et al.* model and to encourage them to reflect on the use of models in general.

The district nurses, although managed by me at Burford, belonged to a wider professional group of district nurses that was actively trying to develop a philosophy of practice for district nursing across Oxfordshire. Fortunately I am able to draw on extensive notes I made during this meeting to enable me to portray the conclusions we reached.

I presented the group with three basic questions:

(1) Why do we use the Roper *et al.* model?
(2) What are its relative merits and disadvantages?
(3) How does it fit in with our newly developed philosophy for practice?

A number of key issues emerged that reflects an overall general dissatisfaction and discomfort with using this model.

The practitioners tended to only fill in activities of living boxes when these were relevant. Whilst this may seem sensible, it created an impression to others that the practitioner had not completed the assessment or did not consider certain activities of living important enough. Part of this difficulty lay with the practitioners not considering the needs of the associate nurses. The primary nurses often had this information in their head. Often the practitioners would only fill in four boxes.

It was felt that the model resembled a check list that led to information being collected in a rigid and stereotyped way which encouraged a functional focus and task approach to practice.

It was often difficult to know in which box to record certain information about the patient. This point illustrates how the practitioners tended to fit the patient to the model rather than use the model to see the patient. This last point has been highlighted by Webb (1986b, p.172):

'More profound criticisms of nursing models draw attention to problems in using them because they are not spelt out in sufficient detail. Several authors in this book have found difficulty in deciding under which heading to enter a particular piece of information in an assessment scheme.'

This issue detracted from seeing the 'person' in a holistic sense. The reductionist feel about the model was reinforced by a lack of focus on social and psychological aspects of the person's experiences. The primary nurses in particular gave a number of examples where they had only seen the person as a patient in hospital rather than as a person in his or her community. On a practical level this had sometimes led to an inappropriate or poorly planned discharge.

Neither had the model encouraged the practitioners to focus on what the illness meant to the patient. In fact the model was felt to be too 'illness focused', based as it was around activities of living, which, whilst useful for functional recovery were very limited for focusing on the patient as a holistic person. In particular, activities of living such as dying, sexuality, working and playing were highlighted as being difficult to assess from within a reductionist approach.

The fact the boxes existed limited the potential to be creative with assessment. The model encouraged a 'one-off' assessment rather than a continued assessment. In this respect much useful information was not perceived or else became buried within 'progress notes'. As such, the model's assessment was felt to be insensitive and intrusive. It was also felt to be inconsistent, with different practitioners interpreting the nature of the activities of living differently.

The overall conclusion was that the model did not reflect the hospital's philosophy for practice. It is pertinent to note that the discussion focused entirely on the model as an assessment tool rather than as an influence on other aspects of nursing practice. Roper *et al.* could no doubt defend their model against these criticisms as largely being a failure of the practitioners to understand the essential nature of the model. This is, of course, partly true. Yet the model does not reflect the essential way Burford perceived its practice, especially since the practitioners had been able to articulate and conceptualize their own beliefs and values about practice at Burford.

Prior to the meeting, I had drawn up a list of reflective questions that might tune the practitioner into seeing the patient within the framework of the philosophy for practice:

- How can I help this person?
- Who is this person?
- What can they do/can't they do independently?

- What are their usual routines?
- How do they see the future?
- How can they best be supported in the community?
- What problems do they have because of being ill or in general?
- How do they feel about being in hospital?
- What is their social network?

I presented these to the group for discussion as a possible way forward to developing our own model of nursing. The response was unanimous in favour of such an approach.

Philosophy for practice

I have clearly stated that a philosophy for practice is a written statement of the beliefs and values of practitioners who work together. As I have previously written, a philosophy is:

> 'a result of an exploration and agreement of minds about what nursing is in relation to the realities of shared practice that gives meaning and direction to practice in the belief that practitioners who share a common positive belief about nursing within the context of their workplace are more likely to give a consistent and congruent care for the benefit of patients.' (Johns 1991, p.1090)

Whilst philosophers would probably shrink with horror at such a definition, it does emphasize the practical nature intended of a philosophy *for practice*. The definition I have given sets out a number of conditions:

(1) It must always be set within a context of practice. This condition explicitly recognizes that each practice setting is unique and that each group of practitioners must determine their own beliefs and values.
(2) It must always be seen in the context of therapeutic work. This explicitly recognizes that nursing is fundamentally therapeutic. Hence, the central themes within a philosophy must always be addressed around this tenet.
(3) It must always be shared by those who work together. As such it is a reflection of collective ownership rather than the domination of one person's voice over others. Clearly domination over others, whether between staff or between staff and patients, is not compatible with therapeutic work.

However, in being sceptical about the nature and value of such philosophies it is necessary to challenge whether a philosophy for practice can say anything it wants to or whether it should conform to some criteria in order to be recognized as valid.

Four factors have emerged (Johns 1989; 1990; 1991) which a philosophy should address to be recognized as valid and which are central to all nursing practice. These are:

(1)   The nature of caring
(2)   The internal environment of practice
(3)   The external environment of practice
(4)   Social viability.

Concepts

Before I discuss these four factors I must first outline the nature of concepts and concept attainment. Each of these factors is comprised of concepts. Concepts reflect and embody in their meaning beliefs about how the world operates, that is, the meaning of concepts is ultimately tied up with the beliefs their users possess. In an ever-changing world, this meaning inevitably changes over time through reflection (Fay 1987).

Even subtle changes become significant. For example, the environment of practice was originally described as the environment of care. Of 'care' is now understood as being just one manifestation of practice. Whilst this risks being labelled as semantic – after all isn't all practice about giving care or supporting care – the use of language does help others to access the meaning of concepts.

Models of nursing are described as conceptual models, or in other words, are made up of a number of concepts which are words describing mental images or phenomena, and propositions which are statements about the concepts. A conceptual model therefore is defined as a set of concepts and the propositions that integrate them into a meaningful configuration that represents some reality (Fawcett 1990, p.255).

The interpretation of concepts within the philosophy for practice is inherently subjective. They are owned by and have meaning for the practitioners. This meaning derives from a reflection of the practitioners' experiences of using the concepts in practice. Fay (1987, p.49) describes reflectiveness as:

'... the disposition to evaluate one's own desires and beliefs on the basis of some criterion as whether they are justified on the evidence, and whether they are mutually consistent, whether they are in accord with some ideal, or whether they provide for the greatest possible satisfaction, all in aid of answering the questions: what is the proper end of my life and thus what sort of person ought I to be?'

Clearly, the beliefs and values nurses have have been influenced by a variety of factors. The general difficulty in articulating these beliefs suggests they are largely intuitive, or in other words they derive from some fused background of experience, of education, of ideology and theory, and of life. This point is important because of the potential conceptual challenge to the validity of these concepts within a definite trend towards concept analysis and clarification. I am conscious of an ongoing debate surrounding attempts to subject caring to concept analysis leading to some universal understanding.

The advocates of an 'entity' approach to concept analysis (Rodgers 1989) argue that such clarification will enable nurses to share a common language of universally understood and static concepts that will stand the test of time and context, and thus facilitate the development of nursing knowledge and comparative research. This is not to say that this might not be a useful exercise. Such knowledge is useful to inform practitioners about aspects of their practice. However, this approach does prescribe a normative rather than a reflective view of knowledge and hence of practice, the two integrated through praxis.

Rodgers (1989) outlines the alternative of the 'dispositional' approach which accepts a dynamic and pragmatic approach to concept development based largely on common usage and subsequent development through reflection. As such, concepts can only be understood and have meaning on a personal level. One practitioner's personal understanding of the concept of patient negotiation will differ from another's depending on their experience. It is useless to merely prescribe the meaning of negotiation to practitioners when clearly this prescription will not fit with their experience.

As such, this approach to understanding and defining meaning in practice is based on the assumption that practitioners are active and reflective creators and owners of their own experiences and hence of their own practice, or as Fay (1987, p.57) comments:

'... creatures who create themselves on the basis of their own self-interpretations.'

Hence, concept attainment is not a matter of telling people what things mean. It cannot be assumed that because practitioners have collectively constructed a composite statement of their beliefs and values they share similar understandings of these concepts. This understanding can only be a 'constructed' process of building upon existing meaning. Kingholm (1991) quotes Hewson and Hewson (1989):

'... knowing, active, purposive, adaptive, self aware beings whose knowledge and purposes have consequences for their actions. They must construct their own knowledge, using their existing knowledge to do so.'

This quote sets out preconditions to being able to do this, preconditions that can be met through guided reflection. Through reflection on experience the practitioner is able to explore their interpretations of concepts identified in the philosophy for practice and which they accept as their own, and to restructure their meanings of these. This is particularly useful when guided through an individual or group supervisor (Johns 1993) where practitioners who work together can share similar experiences of practice and where a shared understanding of concepts becomes increasingly possible.

Reflection shares a belief with 'constructivism' with its basic concern of how people make sense of the constantly changing nature of their experience (Kingholm 1991).

Nurses who are non-reflective are at risk of adopting a formulaic perception of their patients, clients and families. Such a perception limits their potential to see these people as they are; rather, such an approach would encourage the nurse to frame the patient within the formula of the model. Such models do not encourage the nurse to awake to the human encounter between nurse and patient but rather to remain detached from the patient and subsequently from themselves. In the process it will stifle the necessary commitment and passion for human encounter and with it the potential for caring at all. Nursing would become reduced to a series of obligatory tasks done for people. Indeed many observers might argue that this is the reality for much of nursing practice.

If this sounds rather gloomy and pessimistic I do believe there is a glorious horizon that can illuminate this barren landscape. Watson (1990) makes a plea for informed passion which is nurtured through reflection. She says (p.18) this passion is:

'... informed by thought, reflection and contemplation giving rise to moral landscapes and contexts of human and nature relational concerns.'

Without doubt, there is a shifting tide in nursing towards Watson's moral landscapes within a paradigm of nursing as human science. Very few practitioners these days would deny that patients are individual human-beings with unique health needs that are holistic in nature, and as individuals are entitled to basic human rights of respect, dignity and control of their lives. Similarly very few nurses would argue that caring is not central to nursing in responding to the health needs of patients.

Conclusions

This chapter has explicated a number of issues concerned with the choice of nursing models by practitioners. Central to this discussion has been a critique of the 'functional' approach to nursing practice with its compatible view of nursing models. Contrary to this position is the 'reflective' approach to practice that requires a sensible approach to choosing a model of nursing based on compatibility of practitioners' beliefs and values about the nature of their practice with the assumptions that underpin a particular model of nursing, or choosing to construct a 'tailor-made' model, as reflected in the BNDU model.

Chapter 2 considers how the BNDU model was constructed within this approach.

References

Aggleton, P. & Chalmers, H. (1987) Models of nursing practice and education. *Journal of Advanced Nursing*, **12**, 573–81.

Benner, P. & Wrubel, J. (1989) *The Primacy of Caring: Stress and coping in health and illness.* Addison–Wesley Publishing Company, Menlo Park, California.

Beyer, J.E. & Marshall, J. (1981) The interpersonal dimension of collegiality. *Nursing Outlook*, **29**(11), 662–5.

Carr, W. & Kemmis, S. (1986) *Becoming Critical.* Falmer Press, London.

Fawcett, J. (1984) *Analysis and Evaluation of Conceptual Models of Nursing.* Fred Davis, Philadelphia.

Fawcett, J. (1990) Conceptual Models and Rules for Nursing Practice. In: *The Nursing Profession: Turning Points*, (ed. N.L. Chaska). C.V. Mosby, St. Louis.

Fay, B. (1987) *Critical Social Science.* Polity Press, Cambridge.

Hall, L.E. (1964) Nursing – What is it? *The Canadian Nurse*, **60**(2), 150–54.

Hewson, P.W. & Hewson, M.G.A-B. (1989) Analyzing and use of a task for identifying conceptions of teaching science. *Journal of Education for Teaching*, **15**, 191.

Jackson, M. (1986) On maps and models. *Senior Nurse*, **5**(4), 24–6.

Johns, C.C. (1989) Developing a philosophy for practice: Part 1. *Nursing Practice*, **3**(1), 2–5.

Johns, C.C. (1990) Developing a philosophy for practice: Part 2. *Nursing Practice*, **3**(2), 2–5.

Johns, C.C. (1991) The Burford Nursing Development Unit holistic model of nursing practice. *Journal of Advanced Nursing*, **16**, 1090–98.

Johns, C.C. (1993) Professional supervision. *Journal of Nursing Management*, **1**(1), 9–18.

Kingholm, A. (1991) A constructivist approach to concept attainment. *Nurse Education Today*, **11**, 310–14.

Luker, K. (1988) Do models work? *Nursing Times*, **84**(5), 27–9.

Meleis, A.I. (1985) *Theoretical Nursing: Development and Progress*. J.B. Lippincott Company, Philadelphia.

Mezirow, J. (1981) A Critical Theory of Adult Learning and Education. *Adult Education*, **32**(1), 3–24.

Miller, A. (1985) The relationship between nursing theory and nursing practice. *Journal of Advanced Nursing*, **10**(5), 417–24.

Ottaway, J. (1976) A change strategy to implement new norms, new styles and new environment in the work organization. *Personnel Review*, **5**(1), 13–18.

Pearson, A. (1983) *The Clinical Nursing Unit*. Heinemann Medical Books, London.

Pearson, A. (1988) *Primary Nursing: Nursing in the Burford and Oxford Nursing Development Units*. Croom Helm, Sydney.

Rawnsley, M. (1990) Of human bonding: the context of nursing as caring. *Advances in Nursing Science*, **13**(1), 41–8.

Rodgers, B.L. (1989) Concepts, analysis and the development of nursing knowledge: the evolutionary cycle. *Journal of Advanced Nursing*, **14**, 330–35.

Roper, N., Logan, W.W. & Tierney, A.J. (1980) *The Elements of Nursing*. Churchill Livingstone, Edinburgh.

Watson, J. (1990) Caring knowledge and informed moral passion. *Advances in Nursing Science*, **13**(1), 15–24.

Webb, C. (1986a) Introduction; towards a critical analysis of nursing models. In: *Women's Health: Using Nursing Models*, (ed. C. Webb). Hodder & Stoughton, Sevenoaks.

Webb, C. (1986b) Postscript. In: *Women's Health: Using Nursing Models*, (ed. C. Webb). Hodder & Stoughton, Sevenoaks.

Chapter 2
Constructing the BNDU Model

Christopher Johns

The third edition of the philosophy for practice at Burford is shown in Fig. 2.1. This figure includes a commentary on the revisions made from the first and second editions.

We believe:

'... that care is centred around the needs of the patient. In this respect the nurse works with the patient from a basis of concern and mutual understanding where the patient's experience and need for control in their lives is recognized. In this way trust is developed between patient and nurse that enhances care. This extends to the patient's family, friends and others that make up the patient's social and cultural world including their pets as desired.'

The second draft stated:

'... that care is centred around the needs of the patient. In this respect the nurse works with the patient on the basis of mutual understanding where patients can experience flexibility and control of their lives as they would do at home.'

We felt it impossible for patients to 'experience flexibility and control as they would at home'. This was too ideal. What was reasonable was that the nurse should recognize the need for control. At the same time we made the concept of 'the patient's experience' more explicit.

'... that this approach is holistic in nature and for the benefit of the patient, whether towards recovery through rehabilitation, through respite care or towards adaptation with altered health states including death, or towards reducing the impact of stress for the individual and family. In this respect, effective patient care and comfort is the first priority of this hospital.'

The second draft had not stated:

'... or towards reducing the impact of stress for the individual and family.'

Whilst this might be implied in the other words, we felt we wanted to highlight the extent that care was family orientated.

'The hospital is an integral part of community care that aims to meet and develop the needs of the community it serves whether in the person's own home or in the hospital itself as becomes necessary. As such it is responsive and sensitive to the community it serves.'

'... that the essence of care is to support the patient as a person within the community. In this respect, assessment must focus on the patient as a member of the community and be carried out with sensitivity in a non-intrusive manner.'

This last statement was the only addition to the second draft. It was added as a reflection of how insensitive and intrusive the primary and district nurses felt about their use of the Roper *et al.* model.

'...that through its status as a nursing development unit the hospital continually strives to improve care to patients, and by achieving and evaluating this, develops the social value of nursing. We have a responsibility to share our work with other nurses and health workers that enables them to benefit from our expertise and development.'

'... that care given by a community hospital is best given by those who care and have respect for each other..., despite differences of opinion at times, and who can share their feelings at appropriate times openly and mutually support others where needed.... This is the foundation of a therapeutic environment that can only enhance patient care in the future of the Burford Community hospital.'

Fig. 2.1 Burford's philosophy for practice (third edition – revised December 1990).

The development of the Burford philosophy for practice has been described elsewhere (Johns 1991). The method employed to secure open contribution, participation and collective agreement with practitioners involved using large sheets of paper on the 'staff room' wall inviting contributions as to practitioners' beliefs about nursing at Burford. After a month or so, when two sheets were filled and all practitioners had had the opportunity to be involved, the list of beliefs was typed out and a copy given to each member of staff. These were then discussed over a series of staff meetings. These meetings enabled people to discuss the meaning of concepts and explore obvious contradictions and differences.

Eventually the list of beliefs was to become the first draft of the philosophy. This was amended and agreed to represent collective beliefs at a subsequent staff meeting. All original statements were reflected as agreed in the final statement. It is important to emphasize that this was the beginning of a dynamic process. As such, the philosophy is always open to reflective change. The opportunities for reflection are manifested throughout all groups and meetings at the hospital.

Assumptions

In discussing the four factors that need to be addressed within any valid philosophy for practice, I shall begin to make explicit a number of assumptions that underpin the BNDU model of nursing.

(1) The first assumption is that the BNDU model is grounded in a valid or cogent philosophy for practice.
(2) The second assumption is that the BNDU model is a reflective and responsive form in context with the environment in which it is practised.
(3) The third assumption is that practitioners are active and reflective creators and owners of their own practice. However, this is always in the context of practitioners being, at the same time, determined by their practice. By this I mean that being creative takes place against a background of norms and previous experiences that constitute who the practitioner is.
(4) The fourth assumption is that nursing practice is underpinned by the concept of human caring. The particular way human caring is perceived is expressed within the philosophy for practice.
(5) The fifth assumption is that 'inside every nurse is a humanist struggling to get out', (see 'Fifth assumption', below).
(6) The sixth assumption is that all nursing actions take place within the concept of the nurse–patient relationship (see 'Sixth assumption', below).

The nature of caring

In integrating caring into our knowledge to date, it is becoming increasingly obvious that caring is the foundational ontological substance of nursing and underpins nursing's epistemology (Watson, 1990, p.21). As Carper (1979, p.12) informs us:

'Caring, as a professional and personal value, is of central importance in providing a normative standard which governs our action and our attitudes toward those for whom we care.'

It is claimed that the phenomena of interest to the discipline of nursing are capsulized by four central concepts: person, environment, health and nursing (Fawcett 1984). Indeed, so well accepted is this claim that the validity of models is judged upon the would-be model's allegiance to these criteria. Indeed a metaparadigm is claimed. However, criticism of this metaparadigm is evident. Watson (1990, p.21) asserts a claim for nursing to incorporate human caring within its paradigm:

> 'The most fundamental "wide awake" landscape question is how we view person *and caring.*'

A number of discrete caring concepts have been explicated from the Burford philosophy. These caring concepts are shown configuratively in Fig. 2.2. This figure illustrates the conceptual framework of the BNDU model and how the various concepts with the BNDU model relate to each other within the total experience of nursing. The configuration has changed from the way I originally presented it (Johns 1991), although the concepts themselves are unchanged.

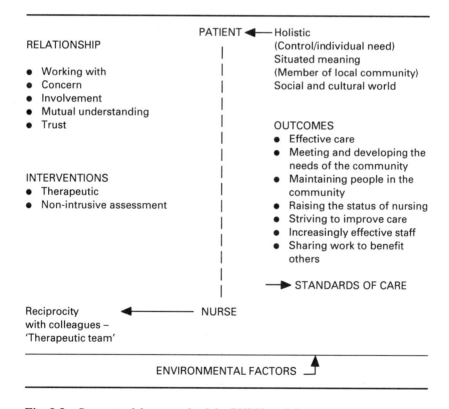

Fig. 2.2   Conceptual framework of the BNDU model.

Caring is defined through the relationships between the different concepts within the conceptual framework. No extensive concept analysis is undertaken for reasons I have outlined previously. The validity of the concepts is judged through the similar use of these concepts by other nursing authors and because they are grounded in practice, or in other words through reflection on experience. As such they are not normative or instrumental, rather they are reflective and open to change.

The similarity with other authors' use of similar concepts is reflected in the use of quotes from this literature. This use does not imply that these concepts have been 'lifted' and applied to Burford's practice as some conceptual nicety. Rather this literature has been chosen because it most reflects the beliefs expressed by Burford's practitioners.

On being a patient

Holism

The core assumption of holism is the recognition that patients are whole people and cannot be viewed in reductionist terms, that is, as parts, systems or mind–body split. Hence the whole cannot be understood merely by isolating and examining its parts (Kramer 1990). Holism takes a view of health as:

'... active, changing and creative – i.e. continually changing in novel ways.' (Kramer 1990, p.247)

In this sense, the health experience is always unique for both the person receiving care and for the care giver. Within the context of Burford's practice these are the patient and the nurse. Whilst they may both have had similar experiences these experiences can never be the same. Holistic nursing moves beyond disease management and requires that the nurse and patient collaborate towards health. Collaboration mandates a focus on the whole person, including the environment within which individuals are located (Freund 1984).

This sense of environment and collaboration is captured by Kramer (1990). She states (p.247) that:

'The holistic view holds the individual ultimately responsible for health, and individuals are deemed both capable and responsible for choosing experiences that will enhance health. In the holistic view, the health care provider is not in a detached power position in relation to the patient. Rather both are active and committed participants in enhancing growth towards health.'

Holism is a word that wraps up many of the key concepts that are found within the BNDU philosophy for practice, for example, 'that care is centred around the needs of the patient' and 'the nurse works with the patient from a basis of concern and mutual understanding.' These particular concepts will be discussed in greater depth later in this chapter.

The concept of holism moves nurses away from seeing the patient within the previously dominant medical model perspective. As Freund (1984, p.16) comments:

'The holistic approach avoids monocausal explanations and emphasises the significance of the 'subjective' dimensions of health. This can be seen as a methodological revolt against medical positivism.'

Kramer (1990, p.247) supports this position by stating:

'Development of knowledge for holistic practice will require not only a departure from the predominant value of empirical knowledge, but it will demand developing processes for creating, representing and evaluating other knowledge patterns.'

The BNDU model is a way of representing holistic knowledge patterns and the critical descriptions of the model in use within this book are a way of evaluating this knowledge pattern. The fundamental position of reflective practice within the model presentation fits with the concept of holism as 'active, changing and creative'. Reflection is the means to such understanding and knowledge and is liberating for both nurses and patients.

People do not live in vacuums; they are active members of cultural and social communities. Within these communities people have networks of relationships and roles with other people, most notably within the family. As people do not live in vacuums it is obviously necessary that nurses do not see patients in this way, but do see them as members of their communities. Hence a 'patient' must always include this network of family and community roles and relationships.

Equally, a spouse is not viewed merely as a spouse but in a similar holistic way as the patient. As such, all the caring processes extended towards the patient are simultaneously extended to the family and others as appropriate. As a consequence the nurse comes to understand not just the situated meaning of the patient but of the people who constitute the patient's significant social network.

Situated meaning

Besides the notion that a person is always more than a patient in terms of their social and cultural world, the patient's perspective on the meaning of the health event that brings him or her into contact with nursing can be seen in terms of their accumulated experiences. Only by coming to 'know' this 'situated meaning' can the nurse understand the perspectives and needs of the patient and hence effectively help.

Benner and Wrubel (1989, p.54) differentiate between the concept of 'situated freedom' and 'radical freedom':

'Situated freedom recognizes that the person is no longer viewed as freely choosing all actions all the time. People are either radically free or unfree. Radical freedom is the modern view that people can choose all their meanings all the time. But this view ignores that the choice of meanings is predicated on the meanings available in the person's own background, culture and language.'

As such, the Burford philosophy statement – 'where the patient's need for control in their lives is recognized' – is a reflection of this situated meaning. Expecting the patient to take control of their life whilst in hospital, to collaborate with different nurses, to make decisions, may become a form of oppression and hence be anti-therapeutic. In understanding 'who the person is' the nurse will immediately put the person into context of what the situation means to the person.

The person may need to be dependent on the nurse. Indeed their physical condition may offer no real alternatives. However, they may resent this enforced dependency. They may need to feel fiercely independent. In either situation the nurse may or may not consider this appropriate. The following day the patient may perceive their situation differently. They may be ambivalent about themself and hold simultaneously contradictory views about their level of dependence and need for assistance.

Similarly, the patient's family may hold contradictory views about the patient's health and conflicting views with the patient. Balancing these views becomes an ethical issue. People do not put their lives on standstill whilst in hospital. Their lives continue and:

'They continue to be engaged by concerns, meanings and even a limited future. They respond as the situation demands and as it unfolds in time.' (Benner & Wrubel 1989, p.15)

Understanding the situated meanings of patients may not be easy for the nurse. Nurses have to explicate their own concerns and meanings from those of the patient in order to see the patient clearly. The difficulty with this is the tendency to always impose meaning on other people's experiences. This of course leads to labelling and stereotyping behaviour by the nurse that is antithetical to therapeutic work.

On the nurse–patient relationship

This last point leads into a consideration of the nurse–patient relationship as the milieu for all caring. It is not easy to use the words 'nurse' or 'patient' because of the non-therapeutic images they create. These images tend to blur the fact that both nurses and patients are human-beings, and as such are responsible, thinking and feeling creatures with their own views and concerns of the world as suggested through understanding the concept of 'situated meaning'.

Hence, within the nurse–patient relationship where one person (the nurse) is designated to help another (the patient) this relationship must be based on a 'what it means to be human' understanding of each other. In other words, this relationship like all relationships, whether labelled professional or personal, is a two-way process.

Despite this concern with images, I feel it is necessary to continue to use the words nurse and patient because they have become so integral to nursing.

'Working with'

'Working with' can be understood through the writings of Alfano (1971). She made a number of distinctions between 'task-orientated' practice and 'professionally-orientated' practice (pp.277–8), a key one being:

Task-orientated practice	Professionally-orientated practice
Predominantly task-orientated rather than patient-orientated. Nurse acts as though she sees nursing as a series of tasks to be done 'to', 'for' or 'at' the patient on a time schedule.	Predominantly patient-concern-orientated. Nurse acts as though she sees nursing as a process in which she 'engages' with the patient and family to foster growth, learning and healing. Essentially she deals with the total life processes in finding solutions to human problems.

For the nurse, 'working with' a patient is based on the holistic recognition of the patient and other members of their social world. In this collaborative relationship, care is always negotiated as appropriate to the situation. In some situations this may not be possible where the patient's ability to achieve this is compromised in some way. In such situations, the nurse strives to act in the patient's best interests within a paternalistic mode.

Concern

The significance of concern is that what the patient is experiencing is important to the nurse as a person. To work with patients involves the nurse in being concerned for the patient. This assumes that caring matters to the nurse. As Benner and Wrubel (1989, pp.86–7) comment:

> 'Concern is a way of being involved in one's world. Concern describes a phenomenological relationship wherein the world is apprehended directly in terms of its meaning for the self and that things matter to us.'

Concern for the patient is not unconditional. The nurse is not a robot who can turn on 'concern' at appropriate times. Rather it is a reflection of the commitment I have previously described as a way of being in the world that orientates the person to act in certain compatible ways (Van Hooft 1987). Yet nurses are human, and, as such, have concerns of their own to deal with if they are to be available to be and work with the patient.

Just as the nurse tunes into the concerns of the patient and the family as the basis for helping them, so nurses must tune into their own feelings and concerns and recognize these as valid. Indeed without this recognition the nurse is unable to care at all. As Callaghan (1987) says 'emotions energise the human quest'. For nurses to use themselves in a therapeutic way with patients, they must be able to monitor how they feel about the patient. If they have negative feelings or are preoccupied with their own concerns then they need to deal with this appropriately so that their own concerns do not interfere with seeing and responding to the patients as they are (Hall 1964).

This is not necessarily easy to achieve. As I shall discuss under interventions, practitioners at Burford have developed this concern and skills through guided reflection. The BNDU model encourages practitioners to recognize the feelings of their patient and family within the context of the latter's own feelings. The relationship of concern with situated meaning is strengthened by considering Peplau's comment (1988, p.x) that:

> 'The extent to which each nurse understands her own functioning will determine the extent to which she can come to understand the situation confronting the patient and the way he sees it. Positive, useful nursing actions flow out of understanding of the situation.'

Of course, this position 'frees' the nurse from needing to conform to some stereotype of the ideal nurse as portrayed by Jourard (1971). Jourard described how nurses don this stereotype when donning their uniform. This serves to alienate nurses from their real selves and, as a consequence, their real selves are unavailable to work with patients' emotional and psychological needs. To see patients as individual human-beings requires the reciprocity that nurses also see and value themselves as human-beings. This reciprocity is a significant environmental factor. If nurses perceive themselves as units of work then they will view their patients in a similar way. This says much about the internal environment of practice which I shall explore later.

Concern also subsumes empathy but is much more than empathy. Empathy is attempting to view the world as the other person experiences it and communicating this 'knowing' to the patient. Hence empathy can be undertaken from a detached or objective perspective irrespective of actual concern for the patient. However, it is more likely that the nurse who is concerned for the patient will struggle to project their own experiences into the patient's in order to try to understand what the patient is experiencing. To reiterate, concern is a way of being that determines how the person will act in the world.

Being available

I have already mentioned the concept of the nurse being available to work with the patient. The significance of this concept to caring is widely recognized. Benner and Wrubel (1989, p.13) note that:

> 'The ability to presence oneself, to be with a patient in a way that acknowledges your shared humanity, is the basis of nursing as a caring practice.'

Ersser (1991), in his study of the dimensions of the therapeutic nursing work, identified the sense of 'presencing' as a key therapeutic dimension within nurse–patient interactions.

Paterson and Zderad (1988, p.14) describe 'being with' or 'being there' as:

> '... a kind of doing for it involves the nurse's active presence. To 'be with' in this fuller sense requires turning one's attention toward the patient, being aware of and open to the 'here and now' shared situation, and communicating one's availability.'

Being available to patients therefore involves communicating this fact. The nurse can do this by giving the patient cues. In this sense being available is more than just a reflection of concern. It is saying to the patient, 'I am here for you when you need me.' Like some other of these caring concepts this is not necessarily easy as the nurses struggle to manage the workload and meet the needs of all their patients. In this sense availability has to be negotiated with the patient. This is achieved through a sense of involvement.

Being involved with patients

Working with patients within the nurse–patient relationship requires the nurse to become involved with the patient and family. The essential nature and significance of this type of work has emerged from analysis of primary nurses' experiences at Burford (Johns 1993a). In particular, nurses were inclined to become over-involved because of their inability to know themselves in relation to their concern. Over-involvement is characterized by the nurse 'taking on board' the patient's or relative's distress to the extent that the nurse's feelings become entangled with those of the patient or relative. When this happened the nurses found it difficult to see the issues clearly which therefore limited their therapeutic potential and resulted in their own distress.

Benner and Wrubel (1989, pp.375–6) point out:

> 'It is an art to know what one can offer in a situation without becoming overextended or assuming more responsibility for the situation than necessary.'

Mutual understanding

The other essential concept in caring is mutual understanding. This type of understanding is a sense of knowing that arises out of knowing the other person, who they are, what expectations each has, and of sharing concerns. This can only be achieved when each person is able to be open and authentic with the other.

The patient is potentially the vulnerable partner in the nurse–patient relationship. It is the patient who presumably requires the nurse's expertise. Hence the patient can be seen as being at a disadvantage in establishing mutual understanding. Therefore it requires the nurse to act to establish the conditions to make this possible. By being open and authentic themselves they can enable the patient to be likewise and through this to establish a relationship based on trust necessary for therapeutic work.

Being authentic can be described as showing and being their real selves rather than hiding behind Jourard's (1971) concept of the stereotyped ideal nurse. It also opens the way for the patient and the family to care for the nurse. Being open and authentic can leave the nurse feeling very vulnerable especially those nurses who are not secure. Clearly, to be able to care as espoused within Burford's philosophy for practice requires a supportive and legitimate environment to work in.

Summary of 'The nature of caring'

The concepts that constitute 'the nature of caring' as the first cornerstone of a valid philosophy for practice have been unwrapped as they are currently viewed as a representation of desirable practice at Burford. To reiterate, through using the model in practice and through reflective practice these concepts are constantly reflected on in the light of experiences of working within these concepts with patients, their families, colleagues and other health care workers. As such they take on personal meaning for the different practitioners and in this process practitioners inevitably come to develop new understandings of their meaning.

Environment of practice

Caring does not take place in a vacuum. It takes place within the context of a practice setting. Whilst having many similarities with other practice settings, it will inevitably have many differences based on a variety of factors that act to influence and constrain the way practitioners practice and make a reality of the 'nature of caring'.

The way we think and feel about nursing dictates our commitment and motivation to caring for people – our patients and families and our colleagues. However, many factors in the environment act to limit this potential. If nurses are to make their espoused beliefs and values a reality then they will need to understand these environmental factors and be able to take action to create an environment conducive to defined therapeutic work. Such practitioners say to themselves and to colleagues, managers and doctors, 'We aim to achieve this, but we practice like that. Why is this – how can we resolve this?'

Hence, the focus on understanding the environment is in order to control it, and in doing so to resolve the contradictions that manifest and which act to limit therapeutic work. This is not an easy environment to create. Nurses practise as they do for reasons which are deeply rooted in systems of power and tradition (Fay 1987). Yet, if the philosophy for practice is to be more than an ideal illusion of what practice ought to be then clearly nurses must take what action is needed.

An important factor is having the necessary commitment to take action. Nurses' beliefs and values must be strongly held in order for them to feel the contradictions strongly enough to take action. This is the same commitment to care. If nurses feel that their patients have the right to be self-determining individuals with a sense of control over their cared-for experiences, then nurses should feel the same towards themselves. The two are reciprocated, or, in other words, are mutually dependent on each other. Another way of putting this point is that the workplace needs to be humanized.

An interesting parallel can be developed with social science. Shulamit Reinharz (1988) advocates humanizing social science. She quotes Schlesinger (1962, p.768) that:

'Inside every sociologist there is a humanist struggling to get out.'

Reinharz recognizes that the major barrier to this emergence is the tradition of social science or what Schlesinger labels as 'the empirical mystique that is the only way to knowledge'. No doubt many nurses will identify a comparable concern as they struggle to take on board research findings at the cost of their personal knowledge. However, this is not the intended point. The point is that tradition is deeply rooted in British nursing and as such it cannot be easily or quickly overturned despite rhetoric from the highest levels of health service management of a 'patient-led service'.

Between this rhetoric and reality lie a range of barriers comprised of vested power interests ready to thwart the most committed nurses. In this sense, the model both enables and encourages the nurse to 'see' herself in the context of her practice and to work towards creating the care environment where the philosophy for practice can become a lived reality.

Fifth assumption

Such is the necessity for commitment in constructing a cogent philosophy for practice, to take action to implement it into practice, and maintain this sense of struggle, that a fifth assumption of the BNDU model is that 'inside every nurse is a humanist struggling to get out.'

The model then becomes a means to express this humanism in practice. The environment of practice is conceptualized as having two distinct strands that constitute the second and third cornerstones of a cogent philosophy for practice. In discussing the external and internal environment of practice I refer the reader to my earlier discussions of these factors (Johns 1989; 1990; 1991). I have tried not to repeat much of what has been written before.

External environment of practice

The external environment of practice relates to the context and function of the particular nursing setting. Burford is a community hospital and as such aims to be an extension of the community itself as overtly reflected within the philosophy for practice:

> '... that the essence of care is to support the patient as a person within the community. In this respect assessment must focus on the patient as a member of the community.'

The impact of organizational influences are less overtly identified within the philosophy. These can be framed as a range of factors that establish boundaries to possibilities. As such they need to be understood by nurses in order to manage the tension between espoused values and what is achievable. This tension can be made manifest through the writing of appropriate optimum standards of care that enable both care processes and outcomes to be monitored. This concept is further explored in 'Outcomes of the BNDU model' (below).

Internal environment of practice

Without doubt the internal environment of practice is a complex world. It is concerned with interpersonal dynamics; with roles and relationships between nurses and between nurses and other health care workers, with attitudes, with skills and knowledge, with how nursing is organized, with how nurses are supported in their work, and with the management of change and conflict. This environment is deeply influenced by tradition and power relationships that limit the possibilities of change merely through rational thought (Fay 1987).

The internal environment is directly referred to in this statement from Burford's philosophy:

'. . . that care given by a community hospital is best given by those who care and have respect for each other within our respective accountable roles, despite differences of opinions at times, and who can share their feelings at appropriate times openly and who mutually support others where needed, reciprocating the caring approach to patients. This is the foundation of a therapeutic environment that can only enhance patient care. . . .'

This statement reflects an extension of the concept of therapeutic reciprocity, or in other words the fundamental belief that therapeutic care between the nurses and patient can only be sustained by a matching therapeutic relationship between a nurse and colleagues. This concept of sustaining the therapeutic relationship is supported by Benner and Wrubel's (1989, p.3) observation that:

'Coping prescriptions all too often overlook the importance of maintaining the caring relationship, because the caring relationship appears to be the source of the stressful relationship.'

It is now understood at Burford that a key learning domain in effective work is being able to cope in ways that sustain therapeutic work (Johns 1993a). Benner and Wrubel (1989, p.3) further note that:

'Involvement and caring may lead one to experience loss and pain, but they also make joy and fulfilment possible. In our view, coping cannot cure or abolish loss and pain. Coping can help one manage those experiences, but coping based on caring also allows for the possibility of joy, the satisfactions of attachment.'

However, there are recognized barriers to achieving this work (Johns 1993a), for example, the traditional hierarchical relationships between nurses themselves and the way nurses have traditionally erected social defence systems to protect themselves from anxiety (Menzies-Lyth 1988) and have adapted defence systems in response to the emergence of primary nursing (Johns 1992). These have been shown to interfere with therapeutic reciprocity. Understanding these factors is obviously an essential pre-requisite to changing them if the beliefs reflected in the philosophy for practice are to become a reality.

Chinn and Jacobs (1987) support this assertion with their observation that:

'Most nursing theory represents the nursing world as it ought to be or might be, which is quite different from the nursing world in which practitioners function.'

Therapeutic reciprocity is a fundamental support system to sustain practitioners in therapeutic work. Yet this is itself dependent on practitioners being sensitive to their practice and looking at themselves in a critical and reflexive way. As such, a fundamental approach to both staff development and staff support has been the development of reflective practice. Becoming reflective develops and nurtures the practitioner's sense of commitment and creativity to give the most effective care. This work is only tenuously recognized within the Burford philosophy as 'the hospital continually strives to improve care to patients'. The focus on 'continually' is critical; it is, like caring itself, a dynamic unrelenting process that becomes a way of being.

Organization of nursing

A crucial factor within the internal environment of practice is how the delivery of care to the patient is organized. Clearly this should be organized in a way that is compatible with the philosophy for practice. At Burford, we choose to use primary nursing because it most facilitates the development of the nurse–patient relationship and development of professional responsibility. Whilst it is not essential to implement primary nursing with use of the BNDU model, the model will have a greater impact where the delivery of care is organized in such ways to facilitate the caring concepts.

Tradition

Without doubt, the tradition of nursing or culture of nursing practice can present a formidable barrier to implementing the philosophy into practice. For example, the legacy of British nursing in the 1970s was predominantly focused on task-centred practice. I have previously alluded to Alfano's (1971) work around identifying 'professionally-orientated' practice norms in contrast with 'task-orientated' practice. Alfano's work is useful because it highlights the cultural chasm that needs to be transcended to achieve therapeutic nursing. Organizing the delivery of care through a task approach is, of course, a reflection of the functional approach to nursing. Even so-called 'team nursing' and certainly 'patient allocation' are merely efforts to limit the excesses of such a reductionist approach.

But as I suggested earlier, revisionist approaches have only a limited effect because they are implemented within the existing dominant culture. Hence nothing *really* changes. The 'task-orientated' approach reflects a concern to manage a workload in a delegated and controlled way. It has nothing to do with working with people to meet their holistic needs. Because all people are basically seen as patients, an orientation to managing care as managing tasks is effectively depersonalizing for both patients and nurses.

Through guided reflection, the practitioners at Burford are helped to confront these barriers that limit their individual therapeutic potential and are helped to work at ways of changing them. This also applies to Burford's management systems.

Nurse–doctor relationships

One particularly difficult barrier is the traditional relationship between nurses and doctors. Traditionally nurses are perceived by themselves, by doctors and by society as subordinate to doctors, yet reorientation of practice around the needs of the patient will inevitably lead to a need to reorientate the relationship between the nurse and the doctor.

The crux of this reorientation is towards professional equality where nurses work with doctors in a collaborative relationship towards achieving therapeutic outcomes. It is probably true that doctors and nurses have different values about the nature of health care and yet I assume that both are intrinsically motivated towards doing what is best for the patient. The doctor's primary role has always leaned towards diagnosis, treatment and cure, whilst the nurse has leaned towards supporting treatment regimens and comforting activities. Within a holistic orientation, comfort is a therapy in its own right rather than an adjunct to medical treatment. This reorientation can be framed within two of Alfano's (1971) comparative norms:

Task-orientated practice	Professionally-orientated practice
Major emphasis of care upon medications, treatment and assisting physician.	Major emphasis of care upon patient's feelings, concerns and goals, and assisting him and family through medical therapy.
Interprets doctor and his orders to the patient.	Interprets patient and his concerns to doctor and helps patient directly approach doctor in discussing plan of care.

Of course, despite mutual recognition by both nurses and doctors that the focus of work should be collaborative towards meeting the patient's needs, the reality is that such issues become clouded in professional concerns about power and control. In attempting to make beliefs a reality in practice, nurses need to understand these issues and learn ways to reorientate relationships with doctors. In the guided reflection research (Johns 1993a), the key ingredient to this reorientation was an assertiveness of purpose and action in interaction and a refusal to be humiliated (Chapman 1983).

Another key issue is for nurses to revalue nursing rather than strive to become technicians, relegating and delegating the caring aspects to untrained nursing staff. The research of James (1989) and Lawler (1991) highlights how the key aspects of emotional work and body work are largely devalued and seen as unskilled by nurses themselves – merely being an extension of what it is to be a woman. Yet as both James and Lawler identify, this work is highly skilled and courageous.

I mention this work because the process of writing the philosophy and the written philosophy can immediately begin to revalue these aspects of nursing work and hence legitimize them in the minds of nurses. Reflection gives nurses access to their caring experiences in such ways that they can learn to value these experiences and learn through them to become skilled.

The physical environment

The internal environment is also concerned with the physical environment in which care is practised. Comfort is a holistic concept and has physical as well as psychological aspects.

The 'knowing' nurse can act to manipulate this environment to meet the needs of the patients. This impacts on all aspects of practice from nutritional needs, sleeping needs, needs for privacy, sexual needs, the creative use of music and arts (Biley 1992), the creative use of complementary therapies, visiting arrangements, opportunities for play, dealing with environmental factors such as noise, smells, fresh air, warmth, stimulation ... the list is endless.

Social viability

This factor is taken directly from the work of Johnson (1974) (Johns 1991). It contains three questions:

(1) *Social congruence* – do nursing decisions and actions which are

based on the model fulfil social expectations or might society be helped to develop such expectations?

(2) *Social significance* – do nursing decisions and actions based on the model lead to outcomes for patients that make an important difference to their lives or well-being?

(3) *Social utility* – is the conceptual model system of the model sufficiently well developed to provide a clear direction for nursing practice, education and research?

The philosophy makes explicit reference to the social congruence of practice and accepts a responsibility towards education and research through sharing evaluated work, for example this book.

Social congruence and social significance

Fawcett (1990, p.256) comments that:

'Conceptual models of nursing provide explicit orientations, not only for nurses, but also for the general public. They identify the purpose and scope of nursing and provide frameworks for objective records of the effects of nursing care.'

The philosophy for practice quite clearly outlines the purpose and scope of nursing although it is doubtful that this is enough to fulfil Johnson's criteria. Whilst the written expressions of beliefs are accessible to the community and do reflect, albeit retrospectively, what the community wants in terms of nursing, even this assertion might be an overstatement in the sense of the degree to which the community sees nursing as directed by the local general practitioners who have rights to admit patients to the hospital. At this level of retrospection the concept of social congruence can only be speculative. Feedback always tends to be appreciative and a recognition that nursing does make a different to people's lives.

More specific aspects of practice are now overtly expressed in standards of care. This concept is discussed in more detail in 'Outcomes of the BNDU model', see below. However, they can be monitored in rigorous ways that meet Fawcett's criteria although her notion of 'objectivity' is a relic of a pre-humanist concept of the nature of nursing which is rejected as incongruent.

Social utility

The question of social utility is addressed in the final chapter when I attempt to draw conclusions based on the contributions made by practitioners in using the BNDU model in practice.

Summary of the four key factors of the philosophy

I have now outlined the four key factors that constitute a valid philosophy for practice (namely the nature of caring, the internal and external environment of practice, and social viability) and analyzed the Burford model in these terms. In doing so I have drawn the conceptual framework for the model. In discussing these four factors I have outlined an understanding of the patient, the nature of the nurse–patient relationship, environmental factors and the concept of therapeutic reciprocity with colleagues.

The next stage is to consider the interventions of practitioners in using the model in practice.

Interventions in using the model for practice

Assessment strategy: the cue questions

Quite simply the purpose of the assessment is to obtain valid and relevant information to be able to nurse the person. Key factors are:

- any disease diagnosis or symptom patterns that indicate medical and nursing interventions and subsequent monitoring and helping the patient with prescribed treatments
- the person's perceptions of their need for medical and nursing interventions
- an understanding of who the person is and their expectations from this health care experience
- a constant analysis of data to determine and negotiate with the person (as able) the focus and nature of interventions.

The fundamental question in considering the format of the assessment strategy was how to tune the practitioner into the concepts within the BNDU philosophy for practice whilst simultaneously tuning the practitioner into the patient and him/herself.

The essential reflective nature of practice determined that this could be achieved through asking reflective questions.

'What information do I need to be able to nurse this person?'

This is the core question of the assessment. The simplicity of this question is deceptive. Because it does not lead the nurse into approaching the assessment in a highly prescriptive way, it requires practitioners who are open to this experience and highly skilled at communicating with people.

Paterson and Zderad (1988, p.7) comment that:

'The process of how to describe nursing events entails deliberate, responsible, conscious, aware, non-judgmental existence of the nurse in the situation followed by disciplined authentic reflection and description.'

This is a useful quote to offer because Paterson and Zderad make explicit reference to reflection and note the preconditions to achieve reflection. They also support the notion of disciplined reflection. This is formally recognized within the BNDU model through a sequence of reflective or cue questions constructed to fulfil the aim of tuning the practitioners into the patient and into themselves within the context of the philosophy for practice. As such, each cue question has been carefully constructed to reflect particular concepts. The root of each question has been described previously (Johns 1991). The cue questions are unchanged from this earlier work except by some minor alteration with the wording of two of the questions.

Being open, described as an attribute of mutual understanding, is not merely an attitude, it is manifested in action. Being open involves being open to who the person receiving nursing is and enabling the person to tell their story and listening carefully to this story for cues. Listening involves all the senses in a non-judgmental and intuitive way, and paying attention to significant experiences shared by the person. Being open also refers to the nurse's own experiences, for in a phenomenological perspective the nurses can only see the other person in the light of their own experiences (Schultz 1972), and hence being sensitive to one's own prejudices and being cautious in respect of adopting any stereotyped notion of 'what ought to be'.

It is through being open that people are encouraged to reciprocate by revealing themselves. This is a mutual process and cannot merely be seen as the patient's role to disclose information about themself. Hall (1964, p.152) highlights this significance:

'It is impossible to nurse any more of the person than that person allows you to see. If we permit him to utilize our freely offered closeness he will not only let us see more of him, but he will allow himself to see more of him.'

Failure to create this milieu will lead the person to use masking behaviours and a consequent failure to disclose certain information (Hughes,

Blackburn & Wargo 1986). The prime focus of assessment must be to recognize and respond to the humanness of the patient in order to establish a working and caring relationship, or what Paterson and Zderad (1976, p.23) describe as a 'lived dialogue'.

The Burford philosophy for practice highlights the significance for assessment to 'be carried out with sensitivity in a non-intrusive manner'. This statement was a response to the reflection of the use of the Roper *et al.* model and a reflection of the major weakness of all formally structured assessment strategies that require the nurse to fill in lists and boxes that reduce the assessment, as I have previously intimated, to a task to be done – to get information – as opposed to a process of caring, and the patient into an object that needs something done to it.

The cue questions therefore which should help in tuning the practitioners into the patient and into themselves are as follows:

- Who is this person?
- What health event brings this person into hospital?
- How must this person be feeling?
- How has this event affected this person's usual life patterns and roles?
- How does this person make me feel?
- How can I help this person?
- What is important for this person to make their stay in hospital comfortable?
- What support does this person have in life?
- How does this person view the future for him or herself and for others?

We shall now look at each one in turn.

'Who is this person?'

The fundamental concepts of being a person have been previously discussed.

'What health event brings this person into hospital?'

The focus for all interventions is related to the person's health in a holistic sense rather than a narrower focus on medical diagnosis and symptoms.

'How must this person be feeling?'

This question aims to tune the practitioner in to the patient's feelings.

This can range from feelings about the health event, about the admission, about the pain they are suffering, about the possibility of death, about finance, in fact about anything. What is certain is that the person will have anxieties about the admission, as Paterson and Zderad (1976, p.24) note:

'Each person comes with feelings aroused by anticipation of the event.'

Equally, the meeting with the practitioner is likely to arouse anxiety. The sensitivity of the nurse aims to recognize and help with these feelings, promoting interventions aimed to relieve the most pressing anxieties rather than pursue a line of questioning that may only serve to heighten anxiety and give the person feedback of the practitioner's lack of sensitivity which may weaken their potential relationship.

The question also encourages empathy. It encourages the practitioner to reach into the patient and attempt to understand how that person is feeling. Empathy is not an easy skill especially on just meeting a person. The risk is always of getting it wrong or as Heron says 'bucketing the wrong well' (1989). Empathy, by definition, must always be communicated to the person and hence becomes a calculated risk. However, uncertainty can always be masked by the use of reflective statements, for example, 'This must be tough for you?' Such an intervention is both cathartic and sensitive and yet safe for the practitioner. It opens up the possibility for the patient to say 'Yes, it is' and invites the person to talk about this issue if they wish to.

'How has this event affected this person's usual life patterns and roles?'

Clearly, disruption of health impacts on normal lifestyle. Knowing this lifestyle enables the practitioner to work with the patient to set realistic goals. This question also creates the opportunity to explore how the patient's health might be improved.

The question is potentially very broad. Where practitioners have previously used other models of nursing, for example at Burford with the use of the 'activities of living' model, this type of structure might initially be helpful to structure this question. This becomes unnecessary once the practitioner has learnt to pick up appropriate cues from the earlier cue questions, for example, 'How has this "event" affected your usual lifestyle?'

'How does this person make me feel?'

This question prompts nurses to look into themselves and confront their own feelings towards the person and the situation. The question attempts to cut across any inclination to labelling or stereotyping the patient. The question acknowledges that the nurse's approach to the patient and subsequent decisions and actions will be affected by how the nurse feels. It enables nurses to put themselves into a perspective necessary to establish a relationship with the patient and to enable them to recognize negative feelings they might have about the patient.

Of course, recognizing these feelings is one issue – they must also learn to deal with these feelings in an effective way in order to remain available to the patient, in ways that do not diminish the validity of their feelings or prompt adaptation into an inappropriate coping mode.

Recognizing negative feelings enables the nurse to seek support or to use positive interventions to convert these feelings, for example, exploring the cause of negative or distressing feelings with the patient through the use of reflective questions. An example I remember well from my own practice is recognizing my frustration towards a man with Parkinson's disease who was very reluctant to help himself. I felt this was unreasonable. I sat with him one morning and asked him to tell me what it was like for him to have Parkinson's disease and how this had affected his life. Such was his story that my frustration was converted into warm and positive feelings to the extent that I was able to be available to him again.

'How can I help this person?'

The role of nurses within their relationship with the patient is based on the explicit expectation that they will extend themselves in a helpful way if the patient needs assistance (Paterson & Zderad 1976). This question prompts the nurse to begin to analyze the information gained from the patient towards planning appropriate interventions to meet specific needs. Depending on the circumstances, these interventions will be negotiated with the person and with other health care workers as necessary. The patient's active involvement in decision-making itself becomes an issue for negotiation.

Assessment is always a continuous process requiring continuous sensitivity by the nurse to changing patterns of needs with the person. What a patient agreed to one day may change the next in the light of the consequences of that decision. Equally the nurse may feel it appropriate to confront the patient with their lack of involvement or expectations of what is possible. Within a relationship based on trust, the use of therapeutic confrontation becomes a possibility.

'What is important for this person to make their stay in hospital comfortable?'

This question is derived from the need to focus on the patient's concerns. It challenges the nurse to consider the environment of care and the particular needs of the patient. This question has been of particular value in caring for people with chronic illness who have well established personal routines for coping and adapting with their lives. Obvious examples are times for baths, use of special bedding, and management of medications. Even the most apparently mundane issues about care can not be taken for granted.

This question has been useful for people who are unable to communicate well for any reason, for example, with patients admitted for respite care who suffer from dementia where it is essential that 'normal' management of care and daily routines are maintained. In response to this challenge a self-assessment strategy has been developed to seek out this level of detail prior to admission (Johns 1992).

'What support does this person have in life?'

This question prompts the nurse to develop background information with a view to developing perspectives of likely outcomes surrounding safe discharge from the hospital or care setting. The question is also aimed at the 'support' in order to determine how these people feel and think and imagine the future, and the help they might require to support the person adequately.

'How does this person view the future for him or herself and for others?'

This question prompts the nurse to recognize that this health experience is part of the person's life and that it needs to be seen in context of the patient's past experiences and future living. The reflective nature of this cue question is aimed at helping the nurse to help the patient and family as appropriate, to explore the meaning of the patient's illness and to imagine the possibilities of the future including death.

This may, of course, be very difficult work. It may involve skilful use of confrontation and cathartic interventions. Such issues are associated with strong use of avoidance-coping mechanisms for both nurses and patients, and raise ethical issues around roles.

This description of the cue questions is both brief and limited. How practitioners have used these questions in practice and the issues that have arisen for them are shared in subsequent chapters.

Being cue questions, they do not require specific answers. There are not 'boxes' to fill in. In this sense they are intended as a heuristic device. However, I have found that practitioners stick closely to the cue questions when they first encounter the model. The reasons for this appear to be a reflection of being socialized into using highly structured assessment strategies in non-critical and non-reflective ways. As a result practitioners have lacked the confidence to be creative.

Equally, they need to become familiar with the model until they can internalize it and transcend its structure in order to see the person beyond the model in a truly holistic way. In this sense the cues access the nature of aesthetics (Carper 1978) by enabling the practitioner to grasp, interpret and envision the situation in order to consider their response with appropriate and skilled action.

This, of course, raises questions about how practitioners can learn to use this approach in practice. The actual concepts in the philosophy have not been a problem with the practitioners because these concepts are both valued and seen as desirable by individual practitioners. In this respect the practitioners are motivated to work within these concepts in their practice which, through discourse with the model's language, becomes understood and interpreted in personal ways that are always examined and developed through reflection.

The assessment is written as a narrative (see Appendix for documentation). A narrative is an unfolding story over time that portrays and gives insight into both the patient's and nurse's experiences. Wherever possible the patient's experiences are captured in their own words rather than just simply the nurse's interpretations of the patient's words. This gives the reader a deeper impression of the patient's experiences and an understanding of the nurse's interpretation.

Nursing actions: the sixth assumption

The sixth assumption of the BNDU model is that all nursing actions take place within the context of the nurse–patient relationship. A nursing action is the practitioner's appropriate and skilled response to how a clinical situation has been grasped and interpreted, and considering the desirable outcome of the intervention.

At Burford, care is organized within the framework of primary nursing although this is not a pre-condition for using the model in practice. Primary nurses have devolved authority for managing a case-load of assigned patients for which they accept responsibility and subsequent, accountability for the patient's stay whilst at Burford, although the primary nurse may seek to extend this level of responsibility for the patient in the community following discharge.

However, the primary nurse only works approximately 20 per cent of the patient's total stay and hence is dependent on a number of associate nurses to continue and maintain nursing in their absence. Associate nurses are independent practitioners in their own right who accept responsibility and subsequent accountability within a clearly defined role description.

Ways of knowing and learning domains

An analysis of practitioners' experiences has revealed patterns of similarity of learning in striving to achieve defined and effective work. These patterns or 'domains' (Johns 1993a) are framed within levels of 'knowing' (Fig. 2.3).

Becoming patient-centred – 'knowing' oneself

This work reveals how practitioners need to unlearn previous ways of working or norms before they are able to become available to work with

Focus of experience	Aim of work
Intrapersonal – Self in context of the environment	'Knowing' self
(Learning domain – Becoming patient-centred (moving towards new norms compatible with defined work and roles))	
Interpersonal – Self in context of the patient	'Knowing' therapeutic work
(Learning domain – Being therapeutic with patients and families: • ethical decision-making • involvement with patients • responding with appropriate and skilled action)	
Intrapersonal ⎫ Self in context of therapeutic Interpersonal ⎬ work with others	'Knowing' responsibility 'Knowing' others
(Learning domains – Giving and receiving feedback – Coping with work in ways that sustain therapeutic work)	

Fig. 2.3 Ways of knowing and learning domains in becoming effective in work (at Burford)

individual patients within therapeutic relationships. However, this is not necessarily easy to achieve. The whole notion of socialization suggests that behaviour is difficult to change even though beliefs have changed. This is because behaviour is both embodied and embedded in tradition, and is, as such, not easily accessible to rational change (Fay, 1987).

Being therapeutic with patients and families – 'knowing' therapeutic work

Three dimensions of therapeutic work in working with patients and families emerged from the analysis.

Ethical decision-making

This dimension makes explicit the ethical nature of all therapeutic decision-making and action. It exposes the contradictions and limitations of basing decision-making and action on principle-orientated ethics, demanding instead a deliberative approach to ethics based on the situation (Seedhouse 1988; Cooper 1991). It was clearly apparent that ethical decisions were made from an interpretation of the particular situation as opposed to a formulaic application of ethical rules (Johns 1993b).

What emerged from the analysis was a series of managing conflicts (Fig. 2.4) that mirrors the progression of personal knowing illustrated in Fig. 2.3.

An example of the practitioner's intrapersonal conflict is their management of time. Consider Mrs Smith and Mrs Jones, two patients under the care of a primary nurse. The nurse's decision to spend time

---

The first conflict
Situations of conflicting values within the practitioner (intrapersonal conflict).

The second conflict
Situations of conflicting values between the nurse and the patient/family which subsumes situations of conflicting values within the patient and between the patient and family.

The third conflict
Situations of conflicting values between the nurse and other nurses/health care workers and situations of conflicting values between the nurse and the organizational context of practice.

Fig. 2.4   Classification of conflicting values within experience.

From Johns 1993b

with Mrs Jones has a consequence for Mrs Smith. The reality is that the nurse has only so much time to spend and hence care must be negotiated at both an individual and collective level based on understanding and prioritizing needs which must include the nurse's own needs and the needs of colleagues necessary to sustain themselves.

In considering previous norms, the practitioners' experiences illustrated how they needed to move from managing a workload based on tasks to prioritizing care based on individual need. Central to the shift in norms was learning to 'let go' of the need for unilateral control of the work environment and learning to trust oneself in working with colleagues and patients.

How the practitioner felt about the situation was a major influence on decision-making and subsequent action. As such, a second dimension of therapeutic work was learning to become involved with patients.

Involvement with patients

This work is concerned with learning to establish and maintain therapeutic relationships with patients and families. It explicitly recognizes the human-ness of both the patient and the nurse and that the relationship is a reflection of this human encounter. To be effective the practitioners had to learn to monitor their feelings and whilst recognizing the validity of their feelings also had to control them so as not to interfere with seeing and responding therapeutically with the patient's feelings.

For practitioners socialized into 'objective' relationships with patients and the suppression of feelings, this was difficult work. New norms to support this work are the overt recognition that effective work is the expression of feelings and fears of being overwhelmed or not coping.

Responding with appropriate and skilled action

Linked to this work is the third dimension of therapeutic work – developing a repertoire of therapeutic and skilled interventions which encompass the ability to respond appropriately to situations.

It is in this context that instrumental research, or what Carper refers to as 'empirics' (1978), and extant theories are useful for the practitioner to draw upon and consider in relation to practice situations. Clearly, where research exists its use needs to be considered by the practitioner striving to respond to situations in the most appropriate ways, for example, aspects of practice such as symptom control, self-administration of medication, pressure area management and wound healing.

These aspects of practice are easily framed within standards of care.

Standards of care are a process of group reflection focused on a particular aspect of practice. The group reflect on key experiences in working with patients, for example, who suffer pain, and in the process tease out significant elements of practice which are then framed as either structural, process or outcome criteria. The process of monitoring and review enable these criteria to be continuously checked out for continued efficacy.

Less 'technical' aspects of practice, for example, perceptions of 'being involved' with patients (Morse 1991), are useful to enable practitioners to juxtapose their experiences with this theory. Yet the reflective practitioner never accepts research on face value. Such research always needs to be considered within the practice context and sensibly applied. Through this process the practitioners assimilate such knowledge into their personal knowledge or repertoire of available skills.

Just as practitioners view themselves as a therapeutic agent, they also view their practice environment for its therapeutic value and respond to situations through manipulating themselves as 'co-extensive' with the environment to enhance the potential for patient comfort and well-being. This understanding of the therapeutic value of the practitioners within their environment responding to the patient is an important contribution of Rogers' science of unitary human-beings (Rogers 1970).

The development of a standard of care of the environment recognizes this significance, paying attention to such factors as the tension caused by the nurse being hurried, privacy, stimulation, noise, smell, cleanliness, tidiness and warmth. A further standard of care was developed concerning the environment of sleep.

'Knowing' responsibility and 'knowing' others

Giving and receiving feedback

Therapeutic work takes place within the wider context of practice which involves the practitioners 'knowing' the nature of their responsibility and 'knowing' others with whom they must work in ways that enable the most appropriate response to situations. Carrying out responsibility for work involved primary and associate nurses learning to be able to give and receive feedback from colleagues about work. It explicitly recognized that practitioners did not work as individuals but belonged to a community of nurses who needed to work together to ensure that patients received a consistent and congruent care.

However, giving feedback emerged as particularly difficult work for nurses to achieve because of the need to avoid conflict within a culture of the harmonious team designed to avoid the surfacing of 'difficult' feelings.

One aspect of this work that became apparent from the practitioners' experiences was how primary nurses often failed to involve associate nurses in decision-making. From an ethical dimension this became problematic if primary nurses expect associate nurses to fulfil their role of following planned care. Often associate nurses would have 'difficulty' with patients because they had not had the opportunity to share their feelings about care.

Coping with work in ways that sustain therapeutic work

The experiences that practitioners reflected on were generally of a stressful nature and enabled an understanding of the dimensions of stress in therapeutic work and ways that practitioners attempted to cope with work. Whilst establishing a new norm that recognized stress as valid, practitioners learnt to take individual and collective action to support themselves and others to ensure mutual support and reciprocate caring relationships with patients. Without a caring working environment therapeutic work is at risk of being relegated to personal survival.

Summary of 'Nursing actions'

This brief exploration of nursing actions necessary to achieve and support therapeutic work compatible within the Burford philosophy for practice highlights the relationship between caring and the environment in which it is practised and in particular the need for effective staff development and support systems. The development of individual and group reflective practice and reflective performance reviews is the response to nurture this environment. Through this work we clearly understand the nature of nursing actions necessary to achieve defined therapeutic work as reflected in the stated outcomes of the BNDU model.

Levels of interventions

When the BNDU model was first conceived (Johns 1991) I suggested that Neuman's framing of nursing actions as primary, secondary and tertiary (1980) might be useful. In fact this has proved superfluous to using the model although the consideration of Neuman's work illustrates the temptation to take 'utility' bits from other models. Not that this matters. The reflective nature of the BNDU model allows for constant review and revision in response to developing practice.

Recording and communicating nursing actions

A key nursing action within the model is the way in which nursing is communicated.

The nursing process

Traditionally, Burford had applied the nursing process, and this is the point of departure for considering the impact of the BNDU model on how nursing has been communicated. Developing and using the BNDU model has raised specific concerns with the continued use of the nursing process in its role of communicating the continuity of care and its reductionist approach to psychological and social needs.

The nursing process has no intrinsic value as the means for individualizing care despite the rhetoric which surrounded its introduction that it was grounded in the concept of individualized care. However, this needs to be put into an historical perspective. Towards the end of the 1970s British nursing was deeply entrenched in a task-orientated delivery mode of care to patients. As such, the nursing process offered a vision and focus for shifting towards an individualized perspective of seeing patients. Such a shift would also require a formal and systematic decision-making process such as the nursing process offered.

Its continued use in relation to the BNDU model has been shown to limit the expression of psychological and social aspects of care (Johns 1992). Nurses became conscious of a tendency to stereotype this type of need and ensuing actions and goals.

For example, consider Mr Bish. He has recently suffered a cerebral vascular accident. The description of 'the problem' is best captured in his actual 'distressed' words as written in his assessment narrative:

> 'I'm I won't be able to walk again. My wife won't be able to cope with me at home. It won't be fair on her.'

A typical stereotyped goal might be:

> 'Help Mr Bish to feel reassured and adapt to his altered health state.'

In this response the nurse has determined how Mr Bish should feel and prescribed what he needs to do. The antidote to stereotyping is always to negotiate the goal with the patient, for example, asking Mr Bish how he would like to feel. He is unlikely to say, 'I want to be reassured' or 'I want to adapt'. He has already said what he desires through his fears. When the nurse feels such desires are unrealistic or inappropriate then this becomes a focus for intervention – for teaching, giving information, giving advice, counselling, confrontation or catharsis as appropriate. In each instance the skilled nurse must choose the most appropriate intervention and be skilled at using it.

To pursue with the example of Mr Bish, the actions to meet this stereotyped goal are also likely to be stereotyped:

> Give Mr Bish time to verbalize his feelings. Pick up cues and respond appropriately.

or a less attractive alternative might state:

> Allow Mr Bish 15 minutes each shift to explore his feelings about walking and his wife.

This example exposes the risk of stereotyping leading to the nurse prescribing what is best for the patient. In both examples the nurse demonstrates good intent and attention to detail. Yet it smacks of control and reduces talking with Mr Bish to a task to be done. These 'actions' could also easily be a goal:

> Mr Bish is able to share his feelings about walking again.

The tendency to stereotype needs of this nature results in trivializing the patient's experience. It also fragments the information about the patient throughout the notes. This makes it difficult for an associate nurse to obtain a total picture of Mr Bish in relation to this and his other needs.

Using the nursing process format works well in communicating and evaluating physical needs or where interventions are of a technical nature. In response to this understanding the concept of Special Intervention sheets (SI sheets) has been developed.

Special Intervention sheets (SI sheets)

These sheets enable the primary or associate nurse to identify a particular patient need and write a narrative of that problem and how they proceeded and the consequences for the patient or family. This is added to over time. The associate nurse is thus able to read a complete account of the issue. Such information is crucial to tune the associate nurse into the patient and help the nurse to respond appropriately to cues the patient offers.

A Special Intervention sheet for Mr Bish might commence:

Mr Bish said to me this morning, 'I'm worried I won't be able to walk again. My wife won't be able to cope with me at home. It won't be fair on her.'
It was difficult to give him attention at that time. I acknowledged this fear and went back to him later and sat with him. It was tough for him to explore these feelings at this time. His wife in fact arrived shortly afterwards. She asked me how he was. I felt it inappropriate to disclose his fears with her.
I left her with him.
Please be sensitive to what he is feeling. If he raises the issue again just be supportive and pick up obvious cues.

Chris, 17 April 1993.

There is no need to break down this 'problem' into artificial and unhelpful criteria of problem/action/goal.

Documentation

The documentation is collated in the Appendix. It consists of a number of sheets:

(1) A front sheet that records personal data – white and made of card. On the reverse of this sheet are listed the core and cue questions.
(2) An assessment sheet – coloured pink
(3) A care plan – coloured yellow
(4) The Special Intervention sheet – coloured yellow
(5) Progress/evaluation sheets – coloured blue
(6) A discharge planning sheet – coloured green. This sheet also lists the process criteria constructed within a standard of care: 'Discharge is managed to maximize patient and carer ability to cope.' These criteria constitute a check list of necessary actions for effective discharge practice.

In addition, a reflective discharge summary is currently being developed by practitioners at Burford.

The use of different colours enables easy recognition of the different forms. They are also more pleasant to use. The notes are kept at the foot of the patient's bed. This symbolizes that the notes are indeed the patient's notes and reflects the philosophy that care is concerned with 'trust' and 'working with' and recognizes 'the need for control'.

Of course, such a policy for note storage is not without its risks. One risk is that of breach of confidentiality or patients reading something about themselves which is unknown or disturbing in some way. In principle, nothing a patient might read should be a surprise. This principle does challenge the nurse to work with the patient in written notes.

The obvious criticism of this policy is when the patient does not know something, for example, that their illness is in fact terminal cancer and it has been decided not to tell the patient this. The management of this dilemma is the responsibility of the primary nurse. They may decide that such information should remain verbal. The ethics of such situations can only be managed within the context of the situation. Like all 'situational ethics', they cannot be prescribed (Johns 1993b).

Summary of 'Interventions in using the model for practice'

The account of the BNDU model has suggested a wide range of interventions the nurse needs access to in being able to give effective care. In doing so the nurse evaluates the effectiveness of his/her decisions and actions through seeking valid feedback. Therapeutic interventions always involve a process of deliberate decision-making within the context of 'what is therapeutic?' and a reflection of the impact of that intervention in the context of achieving desired goals.

Outcomes of the BNDU model

Effective care

Effective care is the primary outcome of the BNDU model and this is articulated and evaluated in various ways:

(1)   through reflective practice
(2)   through patients' notes
(3)   through setting standards of care.

These methods are not being prescribed for use with the BNDU model. However, I assume that the outcome of effective care needs to be demonstrated in some valid way, both to demonstrate effective care and to reflect on the efficacy of the BNDU model in practice.

Through reflective practice

The accounts of practice written by practitioners in reflective diaries and shared in supervision sessions provide a rich narrative of experience. Analysis of these experiences gives systematic feedback on the effectiveness of care and the efficacy of the BNDU model in practice.

This analysis is now being systematically undertaken through formal six-monthly reflective reviews which involve each practitioner writing a reflective review of their performance to share with the line manager. This devolves responsibility for performance and its review to the practitioner.

Through patients' notes

The primary nurses at Burford have a clear responsibility to communicate effectively in order to maintain continuity of care and appropriateness of action. The prime channel of communication is via the patients' notes. As a consequence, nursing notes are maintained to a high standard and enable effective audit to be achieved. The notes are written in the format of the BNDU model which further enables feedback of the efficacy of the model in practice.

Through setting standards of care

The most formal of these methods of evaluating the BNDU model is setting standards of care. Burford has developed a number of standards that reflect specific clinical situations. Examples include:

- 'Relatives feel informed and involved in care.'
- 'The patient is comfortable with his/her pain.'
- 'Patients do not have confidential information disclosed about them accidentally.'
- 'The patient has his/her need for privacy met.'

Setting standards of care is a group reflective process that enables a specific aspect of care to be critically developed and monitored to give systematic and valid feedback that effective care is being achieved.

Setting standards of care is a useful approach to monitoring effective practice within the framework of the BNDU model because it is always underpinned by the concepts within the philosophy and must always pay attention to the environmental factors that limit what can be achieved. Hence, through setting and monitoring standards of care, practitioners come to understand and change environmental factors that limit desirable practice and to constantly reappraise practice situations in the light of new knowledge.

Where assumptions have been made about what constitutes effective care when constructing the standard, then the validity of these assumptions can be checked out through monitoring the various process and outcome criteria. This highlights the fact that effective care is not seen merely in terms of health outcomes. The BNDU model is about the process of care.

Besides the primary outcome of effective care, a number of other outcomes have been identified within the conceptual framework (see Fig. 2.2).

Meeting and developing the needs of the community

This statement is both a reflection of the external environment – 'What is the role of the community hospital?' – and of social congruence – 'Do nursing decisions and actions fulfil social expectations or might society be helped to develop such expectations?'

Whilst responding to and meeting the needs of specific patients and their families who are admitted to the hospital, or treated in the hospital's minor casualty department, or who attend the Day Unit, or who are visited by the district nurses, this statement also refers to a more strategic issue concerning the use of beds and resources.

Taking respite care as an example, 'How many beds should be set aside for respite care?' Similar policy questions might include, 'Which type of admission should take preference?' It is easy to acknowledge a rhetoric that the use of beds should reflect the needs of the local community yet, in practice, decisions about admission are based on a situational analysis with the general practitioners, with the exception of two respite beds being set aside.

Raising the status of nursing

Nursing is the major therapy within Burford Community Hospital. Meeting and developing the needs of the community will clearly raise the status of nursing within that community. The philosophy for practice helps to define nursing practice and gives it a sense of purpose and direction that will demonstrate an important difference to those people's lives which come into contact with it and begin to shift society's value of nursing.

References

Alfano, G. (1971) Healing or caretaking – which will it be? *Nursing Clinics of North America*, **6**(2), 273–80.

Benner, P. & Wrubel, J. (1989) *The Primacy of Caring: Stress and coping in health and illness.* Addison-Wesley Publishing Company, Menlo Park, California.

Biley, F. (1992) Some determinants that affect patient participation in decision-making about nursing care. *Journal of Advanced Nursing*, **17**, 414–21.

Callaghan, S. (1987) *The role of emotion in ethical decision-making.* Hastings Center Report, **18**, 9–14.

Carper, B.A. (1978) Fundamental Patterns of Knowing in Nursing. *Advances in Nursing Science*, **1:1**, 13–23.

Carper, B.A. (1979) The ethics of caring. *Advances in Nursing Science*, **1**(3), 11–19.

Chapman, G. (1983) Ritual and rational action in hospitals. *Journal of Advanced Nursing*, **8**, 13–20.

Chinn, P.L. & Jacobs, M.K. (1987) *Theory and Nursing: A Systematic Approach*, 2nd edn. C.V. Mosby, St. Louis.

Cooper, M.C. (1991) Principle-oriented ethics and the ethics of care: a creative tension. *Advances in Nursing Science*, **14**(2), 22–31.

Ersser, S. (1991) A Search for the Therapeutic Dimensions of Nurse–Patient Interactions. In: *Nursing as Therapy*, (eds. R. McMahon & A. Pearson). Chapman & Hall, London.

Fawcett, J. (1984) *Analysis and Evaluation of Conceptual Models of Nursing.* Fred Davis, Philadelphia.

Fawcett, J. (1990) Conceptual Models and Rules for Nursing Practice. In: *The Nursing Profession: Turning Points*, (ed. N.L. Chaska). C.V. Mosby, St. Louis.

Fay, B. (1987) *Critical Social Science.* Polity Press, Cambridge.

Freund, P.E.S. (1984) Reclaiming the body from social domination: holistic medicine's limits and potential. *Psychology and Social Theory*, **4**, 15–24.

Hall, L. (1964) Nursing – What is it? *The Canadian Nurse*, **60**(2), 150–4.

Heron, J. (1989) *Six category intervention analysis.* Human Potential Resource Group, University of Surrey, Guildford.

Hughes, C., Blackburn, F. & Walgo, M. (1986) On masking among clients. *Topics of Clinical Nursing*, **8**(1), 83–9.

James, N. (1989) Emotional labour. *The Sociological Review*, **37**(1), 15–42.

Johns, C.C. (1989) Developing a philosophy for practice: Part 1. *Nursing Practice*, **3**(1), 2–5.

Johns, C.C. (1990) Developing a philosophy for practice: Part 2. *Nursing Practice*, **3**(2), 2–5.

Johns, C.C. (1991) The Burford Nursing Development Unit holistic model of nursing practice. *Journal of Advanced Nursing*, **16**, 1090–8.

Johns, C.C. (1992) Ownership and the harmonious team: barriers to developing the therapeutic team in primary nursing. *Journal of Clinical Nursing*, **1**, 89–94.

Johns, C.C. (1993a) Professional supervision. *Journal of Nursing Management*, **1**(1), 9–18.

Johns, C.C. (1993b) On becoming effective in ethical work. *Journal of Clinical Nursing*, **2**, 307–12.

Johnson, D.E. (1974) Development of theory; a requisite for nursing as a primary health profession. *Nursing Research*, **23**(5), 373–7.

Philosophy

Jourard, S. (1971) *The Transparent Self.* Van Nostrum, Norwalk, New Jersey.

Kramer, M.K. (1990) Holistic Nursing: Implications for knowledge development and utilization. In: *The Nursing Profession: Turning points,* (ed. N.L. Chaska). C.V. Mosby, St. Louis.

Lawler, J. (1991) *Behind the Screens.* Churchill Livingstone, Melbourne.

Menzies-Lyth I.P. (1988) *Containing Anxiety in Institutions: Selected Essays,* pp.43–85. Free Association Books, London.

Morse, J. (1991) Negotiating commitment and involvement in the nurse–patient relationship. *Journal of Advanced Nursing,* **16**, 455-68.

Neuman, B. (1980) The Betty Neuman Health Care Systems Model: A total Person Approach to Patient Problems. In: *Conceptual Models for Nursing Practice,* 2nd edn., (eds. J.P. Riehl & C. Roy). Appleton–Century–Crofts, New York.

Paterson, J.G. & Zderad, L.T. (1988) *Humanistic Nursing.* National League for Nursing, New York.

Peplau, H.E. (1988) *Interpersonal Relations in Nursing.* Macmillan, Basingstoke.

Reinharz, S. (1988) *On Becoming a Social Scientist.* Transaction Publishers, New Brunswick.

Rogers, M. (1970) *An introduction to the theoretical basis of nursing.* Fred Davis, Philadelphia.

Schlesinger, A. Jnr (1962) The humanist look at empirical social research. *American Sociological Review,* **27**, 768–71.

Schultz, A. (1972) *Phenomenology of the Social World.* Heinemann, London.

Seedhouse, D. (1988) *Ethics: the heart of care.* John Wiley, Chichester.

Van Hooft, S.M. (1987) Caring and professional commitment. *Australian Journal of Advanced Nursing,* **4**(4), 29–38.

Watson, J. (1990) Caring knowledge and informed moral passion. *Advances in Nursing Science,* **13**(1), 15–24.

Part II
The Model in Practice

Chapter 3
Caring as Mutual Empowerment: Working With the BNDU Model at Burford

Lyn Sutherland

I shall illustrate and critique my engagement with the BNDU model through using a case study of my work with a patient and her family for whom I was privileged to be her primary nurse.

Case history – Joan

Joan came to Burford Community Hospital after surgery 'for a few days convalescence', according to the transfer letter which her family handed to us on her arrival. She died five weeks later. She had been ill for just the last three months of her 66 years.

During those last weeks, Joan and her family moved from a position of fear, struggle, disbelief, conspiracy and hopelessness to the point where, in spite of their sadness, they were able to share fully in the experience of death as a healing in itself rather than as a failure.

Her admission to Burford

Joan was exhausted on arrival, having travelled by car with her husband and daughter-in-law only seven days after her operation. Unable to keep her eyes open, she climbed straight into bed with hardly a word and slept at once. Only her tiredness, a slight unsteadiness of gait, and the new incision on her partly shaved head, indicated that she was unwell. As the assigned primary nurse facilitating Joan's care, I sat and had a drink with Tom and Val, while they began to tell me their story. Val did much of the talking, with Tom's tacit acquiescence and occasional additions. The salient points gradually emerged:

'They've told us that she's got a grade 4 tumour – that's very malignant. We know they haven't cleared it all away, and that it may grow again. So they might have to give her radiotherapy. She may not live very long, possibly only a few months. We think she knew it was a tumour before she was admitted to have it removed, because she had a brother who died from a brain tumour years ago. As soon as they confirmed it, she started to go downhill. So although we give her truthful answers to anything she asks us, we're not directly telling her anything. She's not asked much at all.'

After I had asked for the few necessary biographical details, Tom and Val left, taking the hospital's information brochure with them. Having been made aware of the hospital's open visiting policy, they promised Joan they would return later.

By this point, I had spent about 40 minutes listening to Val and Tom, and about 2 minutes with Joan. To what avail? I had virtually nothing on paper, no neat assessment tool filled in with an odd word or two under the headings – 'no-one will read it if it's too lengthy', I thought. Yet I felt comfortable about this. Why? I had not communicated to any great extent with the patient, and I had little idea about her current clinical condition or about her activities of daily living. My experience prior to coming to Burford had been exclusively in the acute field where I would have been likely to have required all this 'factual' information as soon after Joan's admission as possible – 'I must get this assessment out of the way', I thought – and seen it as a task to complete.

I can only answer this by referring to the philosophy and model. By the time I was appointed, both had already emerged as a basis for practice. The philosophy had been sent to me as part of the information I received on applying to Burford, and I had felt instinctively comfortable with it in spite of not 'owning' it by contributing to its evolution.

On first encountering the assessment tool, I had found it difficult to know what to do with it. My initial attempts involved 'filling in' the answers to the questions as they appeared on the printed sheet, and feeling awkward and threatened that it appeared to be expected that I would expose and make myself vulnerable by writing about *my* own feelings. It did not act as an *aide-mémoire* for all the things I needed to know about a patient's physical condition, and didn't, I felt, help me structure information useful to other hospital workers.

By the time Joan was admitted during my fifth month as a primary nurse, I felt much more familiar with both model and philosophy and they had started to become 'part' of me and the way I approached patient care. I no longer had to refer directly to the documents in order to recall their premises, and the way of thinking and assessing suggested by the model was beginning to feel much more natural.

So it was easier for me to accept that Joan's need for sleep was far more important than my need to get to know her and check her physical condition. That could wait till later. The philosophy not only sees the person who has been admitted holistically as 'greater than the sum of their parts', but sees the social unit which the person inhabits in the same light. Val and Tom willingly gave me much valuable information in that initial interview, and the above notes form only an outline of the rich store of knowledge not only about Joan, but about themselves, and the frightening, uncharted scenario they all faced.

At the end of the time we spent together, a picture was emerging against the background of the model that indicated a great deal about what was happening to Joan and her family. The doctor's letter was not needed to tell me about her right occipital lobe glioma, because Val described how the tumour had shown itself – the abnormal sight, balance difficulties and headaches that it had caused Joan – and how quickly it had all happened. So the health event that had necessitated medical care was plain without need for a precise technical definition at this stage.

Her family

It became evident that Joan and her husband, Tom, had a close family, and a largely ordered contented life, with the key members living within a few miles of one another. Their son and his wife, Val, had two children of primary-school age. Their daughter Ann worked in a local shop. They had many friends in the area. Val and Ann's unwavering support for Joan and for each other was noticeable from the beginning, and it was evident that they were prepared to turn their lives over completely to caring for Joan for as long as necessary.

However, this paints too simplistic a picture. They were also upset, shocked, frightened of the future, angry, disbelieving, and desperately protective of Joan. They wanted to explain to me in detail what she could and could not do for herself, and in particular they wanted to control what she was told about her illness and prognosis. Much of their own fear was evidenced in the way they emphasized that she would not be able to cope with the knowledge, that telling her anything about it would without doubt ensure a faster deterioration, and they desperately wanted the staff to collude in all this.

I felt admiration and respect for the way they were all pulling together and supporting each other. I felt that I could help them in the difficulties they faced together with my knowledge of palliative care, and the many experiences I had shared with other families as one of the members approached death. I knew that at that time the first thing I needed to do to help was to enable them to address their fears, which without defusing would lead to a damaging conspiracy of silence which could overshadow and taint all else.

Her care by family and nursing staff

Later in the evening, Joan woke and the full character of her Northern accent, unusual in the Cotswolds, became obvious. Naturally gregarious as a rule, she did not really feel up to chatting to other patients, even though she was quite lucid, and happy to talk about her background and family to me. Not having a great appetite, a cup of tea sufficed for supper, and afterwards I removed her sutures, due out that day.

Her unsteadiness was very evident when she launched herself towards the bathroom. She needed to urinate frequently due to taking dexamethasone. This alone did not control her headaches, for which she was prescribed codeine phosphate at this time. Her bowels had been opened that morning. Once she had settled again, it became clear that she could move herself in the bed, and help with pressure relief did not seem to be needed. She seemed contented to be in the less busy atmosphere that a community hospital can provide, and relieved to be nearer home.

Over the next few days, we found that most of what was needed to make Joan's stay with us as comfortable as possible was willingly provided by her family. She continued to need a great deal of sleep, and her own bedding from home soon made an appearance as she found this much more acceptable than standard hospital provision. All the family and a number of friends spent time with her at intervals during the day, and either Val or Ann would help her with a bath at some point daily. They brought in food she fancied from home, and she began to feel up to dressing.

This of course meant that a great deal of advice, explanation and support for the family-carers was needed from the nursing staff. Problems which needed tackling during this period included careful attention to the nature of her different pains with appropriate pharmacological manipulation, and concurrent intervention to alleviate constipation. Allowance also had to be made for her unpredictable mobility due to the effects of increased intra-cranial pressure on her balance and sight. Joan's mucous membranes became very dry: as she slept so much her fluid intake was not high, and she didn't feel like eating much.

The philosophy stresses that care is centred round the needs of the patient, but also that the patient continues to be a person in their community. For Joan and her family, the hospital became a natural extension of their own homes, and they cared for her themselves almost exclusively, whilst not shunning help from staff when they did need it. The model allowed for care planning which laid the emphasis of care on the family – both as givers, with support, of care to Joan, and as receivers, with her, of care from staff. Far from being passive in her dependency, Joan evidently gave her family much in return.

I felt comfortable about enabling their control of what was happening without feeling that I had abdicated my responsibility as a nurse, with the attendant guilt of not 'doing' enough for them. The best way that we were able to help was by continually re-evaluating the situation in the light of the cue questions and facilitating their care for each other, rather than taking over the caring role ourselves.

Throughout these initial days, the family continued to be hesitant about talking with Joan about her diagnosis. Two things precipitated movement towards more open communication. Firstly, Joan herself began to ask more about what was happening. She began to explore the nature of her illness with me, so that when eventually she asked a direct question during a talk with one of the GPs, he was able to confirm that the operation had been to remove part of a cancer. He stressed that knowing what was wrong would help her to fight it. This was important because at this time Joan was talking very much in terms of the future, when she would be better.

It was hard for the family to know that Joan had asked and been told this, and much work was needed throughout this time to help them through their anger, disbelief and constant search to know what was best for Joan. Secondly, the date set for Joan's out-patient appointment in the radiotherapy department was imminent, and I felt that it was imperative that they should understand that Joan's diagnosis and prognosis were likely to be discussed in full at this time so that all would be in a position to make the best decision about her possible treatment with the staff there.

Plans were made to spend the weekend before the appointment at home, with a degree of anxiety and apprehension as well as eager anticipation. Saturday went well, but on Sunday morning Ann phoned with a story of deterioration – vomiting, increased drowsiness, inability to swallow fluids or drugs – and they all returned to the hospital later that day.

Medication review was not entirely successful, and the following morning also revealed an obvious left-sided weakness. A joint decision was made that she should attend the out-patient appointment the following day in spite of this, and with close liaison and successful co-operation between ourselves, the department and the ambulance service, Joan and her family were able to keep the long-awaited appointment, whilst ensuring an acceptable degree of comfort for Joan in spite of the distance involved.

There was an atmosphere of profound relief when she returned. Joan had been told that there was no need for her to have radiotherapy, and that nothing more needed to be done for the present except to increase her dexamethasone again. Her relatives had been told that her prognosis was only a few weeks, that radiotherapy would not change the course of the illness, but that the drug alterations might help to give a short period of 'normal' life for them to enjoy together.

A further development came later that evening when another of the GPs came over to see her. He picked up cues that she wanted to know more, and Joan asked him directly if she was going to die. He confirmed this, saying that her family knew it too.

Her realization of dying

This heralded a new phase in Joan's care, and the necessity to realign our thinking to explore important issues about her feelings now that this 'new' information had been asked for and received, and the possibilities for her limited future. Although effective pain and symptom control were still of utmost importance, the 'work' that was being done with Joan and her family was much more than this alone. The cue questions, with their emphasis on such activities/words as 'helping', 'feeling' and 'supporting', again helped to refocus our aims to be in tune with the emerging situation.

Tom and each member of the family needed help to gauge how to respond to Joan now that the truth was known and acknowledged by all. There was still a great desire on all sides for Joan's care to be based at home if possible, and yet great apprehension too. Day-time visits home, both planned and spontaneous, proved to be the best solution, with everyone aware that the decision to return lay with them, not us. This gave Joan the confidence to remain overnight on one or two occasions, enabling her and Tom to have time completely alone.

The notes at this time record a number of instances when she had spoken freely about her thoughts and fears. She had told me too that she liked to go to church, and the vicar visited several times. In spite of continuing high dose dexamethasone, Joan's level of orientation, consciousness and ability fluctuated remarkably widely at this time, and this dictated the tenor of our conversations and her daily activity and responsiveness to staff and visitors.

After this short period of readjustment and regrouping, Joan began to deteriorate rapidly. The balance of care shifted as the family members sought increasingly for help with her direct physical care. Joan's pain was by this time controlled using continuous subcutaneous diamorphine, and she was soon completely dependent on family and staff. This situation persisted for several days, with Joan becoming deeply unconscious, hyperpyrexic and tachycardic, with her limbs held in stiff extension. Her urine output was still significant, and catheterisation became necessary to maintain dignity and comfort.

One afternoon as I was attending to Joan with her daughter-in-law, she suddenly 'woke up', asked for a drink, and wanted to sit up. Although unable to articulate very clearly, it was obvious that she understood all that was being said, and was responding as best she could. Some of the family were able to enjoy this time with her, until just a few hours later she became unrousable again. She died the following afternoon amongst her family and belongings in the room which, although a part of the hospital, had truly become a part of their home.

Reflection on Joan's case

Initially there was a sense of disappointment and regret for me when Joan died. I had not been able to share in her final hours as I was off-duty at the time, and that privilege lay with one of my colleagues. Nor was I able to be free at the time of the funeral, although I spoke with the family on the morning of the service. However, in reflecting on her care I did feel very satisfied. Given that we could not change the relentless progress and outcome of her disease, we had nevertheless been able to care in such a way that those remaining were able to continue their grieving from a strong position where their own healing could begin, slowly, to take place.

A review of the nursing notes reveals a wealth of information about their journey in just a few short weeks from a position of devastation and despair, through questioning, anxiety and anger to a place of surprising contentment and acceptance alongside their sadness. There is much comment on conversations with myself and others which charts this progress, also about practical matters and about symptom control, and it is possible to gain a very full picture of the events of this admission.

Reflection on the BNDU model

I am of the opinion that using the assessment tool against the background of the philosophy facilitated what I believe to be our successful care of this family. Prior to coming to Burford my knowledge of models had been very limited, and I doubt that I understood their importance and influence in preparing a practitioner to relate to and care for a person. Coming into contact with the different way of thinking made explicit by the model enabled me to start breaking away from the lip service to individualized care and routinized approach to patients which is so common and into which I had been socialized over so many years. So why do I think this?

Understanding the philosophy

Firstly, the language and format are accessible. There are no words in either philosophy or assessment tool which require a specialist understanding or explanation. There are no complicated diagrams to interpret. Johns (1991) gives an example of how one of the cue questions had to be changed at a very early stage because a problem arose with wording (and therefore a concept) which was not immediately meaningful. He comments too that 'the complex construction of many models makes them intimidating and difficult to use', whereas Damant (1988) notes Baer's argument that a profession needs its own language if it is to successfully articulate beliefs and pass on knowledge and skills.

Wright (1990) questions whether 'new' language is genuinely needed to express new ideas or whether it is only employed to lend credence to academics and theorists. As a nurse whose own education is only slowly increasing, I appreciate it when academics can make their ideas available to practitioners.

However, in spite of this accessibility of language, as I mentioned earlier in the chapter, initially I was at a loss to know quite what to 'do' with the assessment tool. But as I settled into the hospital I was encouraged to find myself beginning to understand how it was leading me to care for patients with a different perspective, even though I had relatively little theoretical background knowledge and practical experience of working out the concepts it embraces.

Because the emphasis is centred on feelings and the total picture of that person's situation rather than on their present physical needs, it forced me to move away from a need to find things out, fill things in and get things done as soon as possible in an orderly fashion. It forced me to start to listen to what patients themselves were saying was important to them, and then to plan care with them from this basis. Duke and Copp (1992) comment that:

> 'The caring aspect of nursing becomes hidden, often among tasks, or defined in the context of tasks'.

It gradually became a welcome release for me, rather than an abandonment into a void, to be able to think through my approach to a patient within this new framework, so that task identification related to physical need was no longer the *raison d'être* of assessment. Although at first I did find myself going back to Roper *et al.*'s headings to make myself feel secure that I had not missed something that was physically important, I did not need to do this for long. Discussion with colleagues and reading about the emergence of the philosophy and the roots of the cue questions also helped enormously in enabling a fuller sensitivity towards the model and confidence in its use.

I said that one of the things that drew me to work at Burford was an instinctive 'feel' that I could work within the philosophy of care. More than that, I felt that it articulated ideas that I had in my own mind about the way I wanted to work with people, but that were very difficult to put into practice in my previous posts. So the spelling out of these ideas gave me 'permission' to try and put them into practice more successfully than I had previously been able to.

Valuing the nurse

The worth and contribution of nurses as persons themselves is not merely recognized, but emphasized as an essential part of the patient's care. Even now, nurses are still more used to acting in a service role and achieving the completion of tasks rather than working in more responsive ways with and alongside patients. The model refers not only to the patient as a person but also implicitly to the nurse as a person. Because the words 'patient' and 'nurse' are not used, it draws away from condemning either to traditional roles. Instead one is led to think and question from the point of view of one person learning to help another – the one with special needs at the time, and the other with special knowledge to help meet these.

Prompting one to think, 'How can *I* help this person' ... how is this person feeling? ... and how does this person make *me* feel?' cannot fail to provoke a response which leads to using not only one's specialized knowledge but also one's own personal qualities and characteristics to help. Pearson (1991) believes that 'the nurse has a right to be honoured as a unique individual as well'. The model gives the nurses permission to acknowledge and value themselves as important persons in the equation, and this has an effect on the nature and quality of the relationships which emerge, and therefore the care which takes place.

Reflection on 'caring'

The word 'care' features repeatedly in the philosophy:

> 'We believe that care is centred round ...'
> '... trust is developed that enhances care'
> 'Effective patient care and comfort is the first priority of this hospital'
> 'An integral part of community care ...'
> 'A therapeutic environment that can only enhance patient care....'

It has also featured frequently in this case study. The model tunes the nurse into thinking about the nature of caring, what it is and what it could become, and thus into one of the major debates in nursing today. It is similar to words such as 'professional' and 'reassurance' which are constantly used but hardly ever defined by practising nurses.

Ersser (1988) refers to the influence of Lydia Hall in the late 1960s, and her description of caring as '*nurturing*'. More recently Pearson (1991) considers the association of care with '*compassion*' noting that both 'care' and 'compassion' are words rooted in the Celtic, meaning 'to cry out with' and 'to enter into'. He also quotes Benner, who in

1985 wrote of her view that 'caring provides *empowerment* (not control)'.

Malin and Teasdale (1991) suggest the opposite – that there is a tension between caring and empowerment. They discuss Griffin's opinion that the very act of caring removes autonomy from a patient. Morse (1991) feels that '*commitment*' may be a more appropriate term to use than caring. She is speaking here of the nurse–patient relationship, and it is impossible to consider the nature of caring without addressing the complexities of this concept too.

These are just a few of the writers who have considered the subject – and wide discussion and a difference in views is already evident. If caring is one of the chief purposes of our work as nurses, then it is imperative that we attend to this debate, reflect on it for ourselves, and begin to make sense of it in our own practice. The Burford model makes it impossible not to do so, for in responding to a person in the light of the cue questions against the background of the philosophy, the debate becomes part of everyday work rather than locked into theory.

In Joan's case, caring for her meant a continuing sensitive responsiveness to the enormous changes that were happening for them all, an opening and exploration of myself and my knowledge into their needs. There was a sense of being available, progressing with them, certainly of empowering them. Joan remained pivotal in her family, and throughout her stay both she and her relatives continued to come to staff for help as different problems arose.

I sometimes wonder how they would describe their experience of being cared for, both then and now with hindsight; whether they would identify with the way I described what happened, whether they would unconsciously use a similar vocabulary, or words that mean similar things in 'lay' terms. I doubt whether they realized that the way I tried to help them was framed by a model, and I don't expect they would give it a second thought. But although I have not formally evaluated their perceptions of the care they received, all informal feedback (chance meetings of staff with family members in the village) indicates that they hold a very positive view of it.

Becoming a reflective practitioner

One of the important things about working at Burford is that it is essential to become a reflective practitioner. This involves keeping a diary as a means of recording thoughts about what is actually happening during the working day. Anything at all which emerges as particularly significant to practice or seems important in any way may be recorded –

interactions with both patients and colleagues, clinical issues, successful and unsuccessful communication may all come under scrutiny.

During monthly supervision sessions with my supervisor, I explored experiences recorded in my diary. In the relating of these incidents, and by engaging relevant theory, I learnt from both the examination of dissatisfying experiences and celebration of successful strategies. These reflective skills needed to be learned and practised, and were not initially easy to acquire, but it gradually became second nature to reflect throughout the day, not just in writing the diary.

I firmly believe that starting to learn to be a reflective practitioner myself has been one of the most important parts of my nursing life. The skills of perception and analysis, the sensitivity, intuition and willingness to be genuine required to be a reflective practitioner are complementary to – indeed, essentially the same as – those needed to utilize the Burford model as a basis for practice.

Reflection on clinical leadership

The clinical leader, in the role as supervisor, plays a powerful part in honing the above skills in the primary nurse. In this case, the clinical leader was also the driving force behind the evolving of the model. As aforesaid, both philosophy and assessment strategy were already in existence when I started at the hospital. However, I was aware that as the person heading up the unit, and as someone with strongly developed ideas himself about nursing, Chris Johns, the clinical leader, had been the instigator of the events which led to the staff writing the philosophy, and the key author of the assessment strategy.

It was difficult for me to ascertain to what extent other staff had been involved, and the degree to which the model was truly the Burford model, or whether it should more aptly be named the Johns' model. Why should it not be? There are many precedents for this – virtually every other model I know of is named after a person rather than a place, and seems to be rooted firmly in that person's work over some years.

It is not given to everyone to be able to study at a higher level, and in any developing field of study there will be those whose gift it is to explore concepts and push boundaries. Whilst not minimising the motivating effect of working with such a person, and the influence that having such a strong leader can have, it is important to note that the nature of practice at Burford obliges each practitioner to constantly look at the work which is going on from their own knowledge and experience. So I did feel able to question those aspects of working with the model which I did not initially understand, learning through everyday events and discussion with colleagues, through personal reflection and through supervision.

Working in such a small unit also means that each person's contribution to the life and welfare of the hospital and all the people involved in it is unique, intensely personal and comes under close scrutiny. It is inevitable that each person's practice will in itself influence and mould the tools being used to frame care.

So in one sense it is the Johns' model, in that much of the background work is his. In another sense, however, it is impossible for the model to be developed without committing it to practice, and so it becomes owned and moulded too by those who use it.

Reflection on the validity of the BNDU model

Another challenge which could be made to the validity of the model is whether it meets the criteria which a number of authors feel should be addressed by any model. Aggleton and Chalmers (1986) for instance say that most models have something to say about the nature of people, about the stages of the nursing process, and about the role of the nurse in patient care. McKenna (1990) found that:

> 'The literature asserts that all models of nursing are constructed around how each nurse theorist conceptualises the elements of nursing, health, person, environment and the interrelationships between these elements.

He goes on to note that some authors maintain that without incorporating assumptions about each of these factors, a framework should not be considered to be a nursing model. Wright (1990), who has himself been the instigator of the development of a model for his own unit at Thameside, also states that models should encompass particular areas of thought to some degree – the nature of the person and their environment, the concept of health and the concept of nursing.

However, he also states that a key element of a model is in openness, so that nursing is not reduced to a fixed, tunnel-visioned approach but continues in a state of slow revolution. The Burford model may not be specific in addressing all these issues by giving *categorical* guidelines within such criteria, but it certainly leads the practitioners to focus on such concepts for themselves and make the outcome of this thought explicit in their assessment and care plan.

Johns (1991) himself refers to some of the published frameworks for assessing validity, and challenges the concept that models *must* comply with a set of rules to be accepted as credible. In writing about practice at all, as Chalmers (1988) points out, there is exposure to the kind of scrutiny and criticism that most practising nurses never experience. This in itself is a test of validity, and along with Johns, as a user of the model I welcome it, despite my apprehension of sharing my own thoughts and experiences with readers.

I have also wondered how important it is to be an experienced rather than a novice practitioner when basing care on a model of this kind with less rigid guidelines than models in popular use. I was certainly glad to have considerable previous clinical experience when I first started at Burford. However, I had not had the opportunity to work in such an instinctive, intuitive fashion, and this is something that I had to learn and adapt to. In the case study described here, I was able to help by drawing on a number of years' involvement in palliative and terminal care.

More recently, in my current post in gerontology, I recall a time when I felt at a loss when trying to help an elderly man with Alzheimer's disease who was extremely aggressive and distressed. I have very little past experience to draw upon of the types of medication and behavioural methods which can be used in such a situation. However, I was in a better position to try to understand and come close to this gentleman in his distress, whilst seeking advice from colleagues to fill the gaps in my knowledge. It may be that those training as nurses today may respond to and flourish in using a tool such as the Burford model, and become effective in their response to people far more quickly than those of us trained traditionally.

Salvage (1990) notes that for those authors exploring contemporary nursing ideology and practice, using scientifically-derived knowledge and transforming relationships with patients are both important. I agree with this and feel that a strong emphasis on the preparation of nurses for their role in its widest sense, but also their continued development, personal growth and support throughout their work, is imperative.

Conclusions

In conclusion, I would like to reiterate that I do believe the Burford model has enabled me to improve my practice by prompting me to think in a way that facilitates a therapeutic relationship between myself and those people that I as a person try to help using my skills as a nurse. Since leaving Burford it has been necessary to use other models currently in use where I have been employed. However, my practice has continued to be influenced by the skills I learnt at Burford.

Case history – Mabel

I became aware of this particularly vividly one day during my district nurse training. I was asked to assess Mabel, an elderly lady who had multiple medical problems complicated by difficult social circumstances. On the day I made my first visit, I was feeling low and unconfident in myself, and my own concerns were still uppermost in my mind as I knocked on her door. Meeting this very agitated and unwell lady for the first time in her own home, crowded with the paraphernalia associated with an extended family across the generations living in too small a space, threw me completely.

My first instinct was to find an excuse to leave and try to get some help for me! My second was to reach for a tight assessment structure with which I could marshall some sense and order out of the muddled situation, and gain some sort of control. I wanted to be told specific problems for which I felt safe to prescribe definitive actions. However, my socialization as a nurse prevented me from giving in to the first option, and I felt instinctively that the second would crush Mabel rather than succeed in finding out what was really bothering her.

So I tried to concentrate on her story, and as I did so I felt my feelings of helplessness diminish as I paid attention to what she was trying to articulate. I slowly began to think more rationally – 'Who is this person? What do I need to know to be able to help her?' As I continued to listen, actively now and with renewing confidence, the familiar cue questions formed the background to the way I began to respond to her, and I found I was engaged in 'using' the Burford model. I know that the Burford model will be helping me to nurse for many years to come.

References

Aggleton, P. & Chalmers, H. (1986) Model choice. *Senior Nurse*, **5**, (5/6), 18–20.

Chalmers, H. (1988) Choice. In: *Choosing a Model*: Caring for patients with cardio-vascular and respiratory disorders, (ed. H. Chalmers). Edward Arnold Publishers, London.

Damant, M. (1988) Innovations in assessment. *Journal of District Nursing*, **6**(9), 9–12.

Duke, S. & Copp, G. (1992) Hidden nursing. *Nursing Times*, **88**, (17), 40–42.

Ersser, S. (1988) Nursing beds and nursing therapy. In: *Primary Nursing – Nursing in the Burford and Oxford Nursing Development Units*, (ed. A. Pearson). Croom Helm, London.

Johns, C.C. (1991) The Burford Nursing Development Unit holistic model of nursing practice. *Journal of Advanced Nursing*, **16**, 1090–98.

Malin, N. & Teasdale, K. (1991) Caring versus empowerment: considerations for nursing practice. *Journal of Advanced Nursing*, **16**, 657–62.

McKenna, H. (1990) Which model? *Nursing Times*, **86**, (25), 50–52.

Morse, J. (1991) Negotiating commitment and involvement in the nurse–patient relationship. *Journal of Advanced Nursing*, **16**, 455–68.

Pearson, A. (1991) Taking up the challenge: the future for therapeutic nursing. In: *Nursing as Therapy*, (eds R. McMahon & A. Pearson). Chapman & Hall, London.

Roper, N., Logan, W.W. & Tierney, A.J. (1980) *The Elements of Nursing*. Churchill Livingstone, Edinburgh.

Salvage, J. (1990) The theory and practice of the 'new' nursing. *Nursing Times*, **85**, (4), 42–5.

Wright, S. (1990) Useless theory or aids to practice? In: *Models for Nursing 2*, (eds B. Kershaw & J. Salvage). Scutari Press, Harrow, Middlesex.

Editor's commentary

Lyn Sutherland's case study draws out her family- and community-orientation to caring. She relates closely to the patient and the family's medical management and she liaises with the general practitioner and the acute unit in a collaborative role as well as in an advocate and empowering role for the patient and her family.

The case study is also an account of Lyn's own empowerment, of finding herself through the simultaneous freedom and support that the BNDU model offers and of the satisfaction she found through this work. Empowerment is a reciprocal process. Without feeling empowered themselves, practitioners cannot enable their patients to feel empowered or act as their advocate.

As Lyn mentions it is indeed a privilege to care for families at such times of sorrow. Yet Lyn is not stressed by this; in fact, as her work progressed she found great satisfaction in working with the family. I feel this is because she has become personally involved and caring has become a mutual process. Lyn emphasizes the significance of the model in tuning herself into both her own and the patient's feelings. Indeed, as I demonstrated in the first two chapters, it becomes impossible to care without this recognition and validation of mutual feelings. It is the failure to acknowledge oneself as human that limits the nurse's therapeutic potential and does harm to both the nurse and the patient.

Lyn only worked at Burford for one year, but she notes how the model remained an influence in her later work as a district nurse. However, when I asked her why she did not use the BNDU model in her district nursing, she replied that she was expected to use another model irrespective of its value in seeing and working with patients. This illustrates how practice settings impose models on practitioners. Part of this dilemma was due to the fact that her district nursing practice had not been defined and hence neither practice nor the use of a nursing model had direction or sense.

This chapter demonstrates how the model can only live through its use by practitioners and that practitioners need to own the model for it to be meaningful to them. This emphasizes the difference between a prescriptive model – and hence the practitioner accepts it as normative – and a reflective model – and hence the practitioner uses the model reflexively in order to interpret it and make personal sense of it.

Lyn's experience demonstrates the prescriptive and normative power of models as she clings to previous learnt assessment strategies to see the patient. Yet she realizes the limitations of the Roper *et al.* model to 'see' the person. It is worth mentioning that Lyn had been a senior sister prior to coming to Burford and as such presumably would have had considerable influence on the use of a model for practice had she then known about nursing models and their use.

It is also important to clarify Lyn's commitment to caring. It was not easy for her to adjust to work at Burford after her previous role and she was deeply entrenched in hierarchical and controlling methods which created initial conflict between her and other staff. But through supervision she was able to adapt to the more holistic nature of the BNDU model.

Chapter 4
Discovering the Art of Nursing: Using the BNDU Model at Burford

Roger Cowell

'We must come down from our position as "objective observers", and meet our patients face-to-face: we must meet them in a sympathetic and imaginative encounter; for it is only in the context of such collaboration, a participation, relation, that we can hope to learn anything about how they are.' (Sacks 1990, pp.7–8)

Reflections

I remember being very excited about showing Chris Johns the excerpt quoted above from the book '*Awakenings*', following an early supervision session with him at Burford. It seemed to accord closely with the way I wanted to nurse, the relationship I wanted to achieve with my patients and colleagues, and with the philosophy and model for nursing practised at Burford. I had been in my new post for ten days.

In my diary I had reflected on a number of particular patients.

Case study – 'Mounty' Mountain and her family

What are her hopes and fears for the future?
What are the family's hopes and fears?
'Mounty' has said repeatedly she is afraid of falling. This is wholly understandable – it is the fear of an unknown future; not one that is allayed easily. Mounty's family fear for the times they can't be with her when she is at home alone.
My words for what help they may need: confidence; multiple supports.
There are no absolute guarantees of safety.
Does a fear of falling mask other fears, e.g. illness, dependence, death?

Case study – Wilfred Turnball

Of Wilfred Turnball, a man who had suffered a number of debilitating strokes, who could only communicate in a very limited way, and who had been in the hospital for several months, I wrote:

> He seems to have an up day or part of a day – when he is awake and alert, eats, drinks and shows an interest in his surroundings and the people in it. Then part way through a day, or for a whole day or two, from morning to night, he is drowsy or asleep, uninterested in food, drink, people or in his environment. It's as if he doesn't have enough energy for every day, and has to conserve his energy and re-charge himself.
> Other staff have told me how he used to be, but it is hard to grasp.
> I have talked only once with Iris, his wife. She seems quite diffident. I think I would like to know how she feels about being with Wilfred as he is, and what her hopes and fears of the future are.
> It must be *very* difficult to visit someone you care for, and who cares for you, and find the connections so hard to maintain.

Frankly, in my early days at Burford, I struggled to grasp and make sense of the model in my relationships. I had read books with related approaches such as '*Awakenings*', as quoted above, and Carl Rogers writing about the therapeutic relationship. Now, more than a year later, I remain engaged in that struggle but from a different perspective.

This new perspective is captured by the following quotation of Maynard Keynes in his '*Preface to General Theory*':

> 'The very difficulty lies not in the new ideas but in escaping from the old ones, which ramify, for those brought up as most of us have been, into every corner of our minds.' (Sacks 1990, p. xiv)

In my early days, I also noted in my diary:

> 'Where am I with my colleagues?
> We don't know each other well enough to be much more than a harmonious team, that is, we are not yet giving each other much feedback – that I want to get and give ...'

I also reflected on my assessment of patient care and tentative use of the cue questions within the holistic model:

> 'These are hard to grasp in that in a large acute ward the principal questions are for priorities of physical care, where psychological and social need are almost identified by chance. It's hard not to ask questions to patients directly rather than bear the questions in mind as cues ... in my previous practice I reflected on my practice more than

many of my colleagues but, in comparison with now, that was not very much!'

'Escape'

The turning point in my 'escape story', the escape from old ideas, was a very painful afternoon of 'group reflection' with my colleagues. They told me that they perceived me as being unsupportive and unforthcoming of feedback. That night I noted in my reflective diary:

'What do I feel tonight?

- distress
- sorrow
- loss
- pain
- isolation
- dislocation
- threat
- dismay
- sadness
- threat
- insecurity
- puzzlement'.

I recognized then that my 'low mood' about myself was getting in the way of giving and receiving feedback with both my patients and colleagues. This cathartic experience made it possible for me to ask more or less the same questions *of myself* as the model's cue questions, to enable me to confront myself – 'who am I?' – which proved to be essential to enable me to nurse my patients effectively.

Illustrating the model in practice

I am going to illustrate my engagement with the BNDU model in practice through a series of case studies that bring out key personal factors in my use of this model.

Case study – Madge Brown: facilitating shifts in attitudes to promote care of a 'difficult' patient

My first response to Madge was sheer panic. She arrived at the hospital on a Friday afternoon. She was far more dependent than I had antici-pated from conversations with nurses from her referring hospital. She was 73, nearly blind, an insulin-dependent diabetic, heavy, with both legs amputated just below the knee, had recently suffered a stroke that had left her with a dense left hemiplegia, and had recently been diagnosed with carcinoma of the rectum.

I felt she would require more nursing attention than we could give so after making this judgement I informed her GP what I and my colleagues felt. He responded very personally: 'Are you saying you can't cope, that you haven't got enough staff?' I said we did not have appropriate resources to care for her and could not see what the outcome could be. The GP replied, 'That's your problem not mine.'

A number of other staff expressed their opinion that it was 'ridiculous' for us to look after her and inappropriate for her to be in a community hospital. That was also my opinion at first but the GP's stinging response to my request for support spurred me to look at this person as a human-being not just as an unwelcome burden on the work-load.

Obviously physical resources such as the use of a 'pegasus' mattress, a hoist and sling made the management of Madge's care possible, even if still time-consuming. But it was the establishment of relationships with Madge and her husband, Bill, which led me and eventually my colleagues to define and achieve desirable outcomes of care, prompted by the cues within the BNDU model.

As a primary nurse I am care-giver and care-planner. As such, my assessment is not merely a snapshot on admission but something continuous, reminiscent of Sacks' 'sympathetic and imaginative encounter'. So it was that whilst giving direct care – assisting her with breakfast one morning – I broke through to Made 'face-to-face'.

I wondered aloud if she would like to take the beaker of tea herself, take her cereal spoon and her slices of toast from the plate. Her poor eyesight required my instruction where to feel for the food, whether she had filled her spoon, where her beaker was and where she could find the plate of toast, so it did not mean I could attend to somebody else. But it did mean that Made was shown that she could still do things which neither the staff at her previous hospital nor her family had let her do.

It was the BNDU model that prompted my questioning, 'How did Madge feel?' I asked her what it was like to use utensils now. She smiled and said, 'It makes me feel human again.'

It is during the everyday giving of such personal care that the BNDU model brings the cue questions repeatedly to mind. This was evident in another experience of working with Madge, when a care assistant and I were helping Madge to change her position in bed one day. I asked her to move her legs to one side. She replied immediately, 'You mean my stumps.' I challenged her with the suggestion that her legs were still legs, regardless of being partially amputated.

Such individual interactions do not necessarily affect the interactions of colleagues even if recorded. It was necessary to communicate the desired outcomes to Madge's family and my colleagues, in a form that might facilitate their reflections on their relationship with Madge. In effect, I was asking them to answer the core question of the BNDU model by rephrasing cue questions in relation to specific aspects of care.

How did I go about this and how effective was it?

I prepared a Special Intervention (SI) sheet describing the two incidents outlined above and asking my colleagues to consistently follow my approach with utensils and to challenge Madge when she made comments suggesting low self-esteem. I asked my colleagues for feedback on how they felt when Madge made negative comments, and how they responded to her. These were both recorded and given verbally.

After a few weeks Madge was referring spontaneously and consistently to her legs and talking more with the nursing staff. Staff, including those who had been critical and sceptical of my decision to accept her for our care, made comments to me on their enjoyment of caring for Madge and their pleasure when Madge managed particularly well with some aspects of self-care.

Continuing assessment with the BNDU model

An individual's health events evolve, of course, and our relationship with Madge and her husband was no exception. Bill was determined to care for her at home, and, despite the limited availability of community care staff and resources, despite the obstruction and scepticism of some community personnel, and despite the added complication of 'cross-border' referral (Madge's GP was in Oxfordshire but her home was in Gloucestershire), a workable package was negotiated. Madge was discharged and her and Bill's desire to be together was achieved.

How did this person feel about the future?

My experience at Burford has pressed me further to support patients and their carers who express a wish to achieve specific desired goals. In my relationship with Madge and Bill Brown, the first goal was for Madge to go home. I was able to monitor the effectiveness of our negotiated decision with a post-discharge home visit, and by maintenance of a flexible respite care policy for them.

Seeing Madge in her bedroom, in a hospital bed, with radio, television and bedside telephone, near a window where she could hear birds outside, confirmed for me that her discharge was a success. Bill was coping well at the time, though Penny Lane, the district nurse, who spent an hour or more daily with Madge, found it a severe burden on her workload.

Respite care varied from four to eight weeks between one week admissions. As her carcinoma spread she experienced greater pain with insomnia and increased confusion and anxiety. Despite medication adjustments she became agitated and suspicious of others. She was also intermittently unaware of whether she was at home or in hospital.

At this time I asked Madge how she saw the future. She said, 'I don't think about it; it's too painful.'

It was also upsetting for Bill and for myself and my colleagues who felt that this Madge was not the same Madge Brown we used to know. The BNDU model makes practitioners continually focus on themselves as individuals, and in this situation made me focus my concern and my colleagues' concerns on our feelings:

'How must this person be feeling?'
'How does this person make me feel?'

In response to these cues, I discussed my perceptions of change with the associate nurses, care assistants, the district nurse and with Bill, so that we could share how we felt about Madge and reach some understanding of how best to care for her and support each other. It felt like grieving.

My care planning became a collegial issue – stemming from the belief within our hospital philosophy that recognizes that we are committed to involvement with our patients and to each other. Rather than running away from these uncomfortable feelings, the model cues us to pay attention to the personal issues so that we may deal with them as significant determinants in the care we are able to give.

At times I was confronted by my colleagues with our difficulties in caring for Madge and this sometimes 'anguished' reflection on our care prompted me to continually anticipate Bill and Madge's future needs.

Supporting Bill became even more important in the light of these changes in Madge's condition and I was able to give him opportunities to share with me his feelings and thoughts of Madge and the future, and how he was managing the meaning of the changes that were happening to Madge. Additionally I suggested that if he decided he could no longer manage looking after Madge at home, then she could come to Burford for continuing terminal care. He was not sleeping much and felt very tired and stressed, but he was determined to care for Madge at home until she died and in that he succeeded.

I feel certain that the BNDU model's cue questions were a constant challenge to Bill and Madge's care and facilitated this process of reflection and anticipation.

Case study – Johny Arthur: the BNDU model leading to a holistic portrait of a person

The BNDU model has also facilitated me in forming therapeutic relationships with some patients in such a way that I can see them as rounded individuals rather than as 'types', which I believe is how I, in common with many colleagues, saw many patients in previous nursing practice environments. To some extent, this may be as a result of a close and continuing relationship, but in my experience, my commitment to a holistic philosophy and ensuing model for practice brings me naturally to reflect on my patients and their humanity.

This is illustrated with clarity in the development of my skills in portraying people on paper, as in my discharge letter for Johny Arthur to his new nursing home.

Mr Arthur was admitted to us for overnight observation, and it was clear that he had a cerebral vascular accident, or at best, a transient ischaemic attack. Over the following few days, Johny was very agitated and restless, and then deteriorated markedly, but made a further recovery in consciousness. He exhibited a severe visual impairment – a right hemianopia – which is in no sense resolved and which remains a puzzle and a source of anxiety to him.

According to his former landlady, Johny has been restless, anxious and agitated as long as she has known him, and these traits have been magnified by his stroke. At times, both in the early post incident period and in the weeks and months since, he has been so agitated as to require major tranquillizers. He responds to calm, firm direction perhaps as a result of a military wartime experience, or, failing that, he may be best just left to his own devices to calm down. It may be useful for you to know that he can be very variable in mood and response during each day and from day to day.

Johny has in many ways made a fine recovery physically. Sadly, however, Johny's anxiety has been accompanied by a tendency to talk quite extravagantly and inappropriately, and at great length. Sometimes he is painfully aware that he is talking nonsense, and it may be interspersed with genuine sense, and he may respond in a fully appropriate manner.

Johny had little or no insight into his illness for a long period of his stay with us, and this was at times a hindrance to his recovery and sometimes, in a sense, a kindness. But he has developed insights which are quite real and deep – for an example see the photocopied Special Intervention sheet (see Fig. 4.1).

It has not always been easy to support and care for Johny. At times it has been pleasant and at times frustrating, difficult and sad. Here is a man whose life has been changed dramatically by this change to his health and our responsibility has been to provide the best possible care and support for him in varying ways in which he has needed it. I hope you will be able to accept him and value him as a person, a man of considerable depth, wit and charm, with many other facets – in short, a human-being like us all.

Special Intervention Sheet

SI 1: Reflecting with Johny on his future

28/2/92

Johny said to me today:

" I don't know why you bother:
I've got no future."

Questions:

When Johny makes such comments
how do you respond?

Can we spend time with him to show
that we value him as a person?

NAME Johny Arthur   PRIMARY NURSE Roger

Fig. 4.1 Excerpt from Johny Arthur's Special Intervention sheet.

When I shared this letter with colleagues they told me that I captured the essence of Johny's essence and care. I contrasted this with what I associate as 'standard' discharge letters which say something like 'Thank you for taking this pleasant gentleman.'

I prepared this portrait from the perceptive and detailed observations and reflections in Johny's notes. The use of narrative form for assessment detail and Special Intervention sheets for particular psycho-social aspects of care gives access to a rich description and critical evaluation of care processes. Learning to observe and write in such ways fundamentally leads to new ways of talking and writing about patients that naturally reflects their humanness as Johny's discharge letter illustrates.

Case study – Aaron Maclean: a puzzle unsolved

Of course, using the BNDU model is not a guarantee in itself that desired outcomes will be attained. It is the nature of the 'messy lowlands' of clinical practice (Schon 1983) that there will be people and situations which, with whatever will and resources are gathered, remain a painful puzzle. This is a difficult admission to make and yet a consequence of my reflective and self-critical nature. This case study is concerned with just such a patient.

At the time, I felt anxious and frustrated to an extreme degree, and even now, months later, reflecting on my involvement with Aaron is scarcely more comfortable. In part this is because I have high expectations of myself, but I do wonder how using the BNDU model may bring to the surface a practitioner's suppressed anxieties and doubts about competence. Such speculation leads me to suggest that the use of such a holistic practice model as the BNDU model may require practitioners to enter into supervised reflective practice to enable them 'to retain control of their work' (Johns 1990, p.892).

I discussed Aaron at length under supervision on about six occasions. When I first shared an experience concerning him I gave my supervisor a sketch of him which included:

> I've got a patient at the moment who is quite a puzzle to us all ... with reduced mobility, chronic constipation, lethargy, low motivation – he sees no point in eating, drinking, in fact doing anything ... he doesn't want to listen to people – if you persist he gets quite irritated. He also requires help – two nurses to transfer him from bed to chair. He grabs people and objects. When you insist, he does stand better, but then panics after a few minutes. I haven't had time to spend a long time with him, but I feel I have got to get down to what he wants and how to achieve that.

Justifiably my supervisor challenged me on the statement 'I haven't got time'. I replied, 'I know I need to make time – I know it's bothering me.'

The question of 'making time' is one which is crucial to me in using the BNDU model in my practice. Just after one Christmas, I returned from holiday to find the hospital nearly full with very dependent people with substantial needs. Minimal assessments, mainly of physical aspects of care, had been made. I wrote about this in my diary, feeling depressed and angry. (At the time I was the only primary nurse):

> 'I met each patient in giving them care, but was able to plan care only for essential physical requirements. I wanted to take time to reflect on the cue questions... *Now* – 48 hours later – I have got up-to-date with physical problems and I know I can communicate the emotional problems and needs, but I haven't put these onto paper. *Time* is a key.
>
> Interventions and evaluation have taken all my time, but now I'll have to work on holistic assessment. Alternatively I could have spent yet more of my own time to reflect on Aaron's psycho-social needs, and how these might have been better identified and met by other practitioners. *But* I rationalized – it does not seem a realistic use of my time, given the pressures of physical requirements – and I have maintained and promoted safety and recovery.'

As I write now, this seems more like crisis management than holistic care.

Returning to the case study of Aaron, I commented to an associate nurse that I did not understand how Aaron 'worked'. In response the associate nurse admitted to being 'baffled' by him. I felt I was beginning to blame myself for this situation.

'Blame' is an interesting concept – I used it in a wider sense than the dictionary definition of 'to fix the responsibility on...' (Concise Oxford Dictionary 1982, p.93). As the primary nurse, I was aware of my responsibility for Aaron's care, but I was also *uneasily* aware that I had crossed over the line of responsibility for my actions to take up responsibility for Aaron's actions. It was as if I believed that there was a secret key to his actions, and if I engaged sufficiently deeply with him, I would find the key, and enable him to resolve his anxieties, take control of his physical problems and get up and go.

I said I was 'beginning' to blame myself. To qualify this movement to tacit responsibility for Aaron's actions, I wish to demonstrate that 'involvement' with a patient, prompted by the BNDU model, may emerge as a slow realization of what is happening in a particular situation.

A risky discharge home – unresolved conflict with a district nurse

Aaron Maclean had expressed a wish to go home, and I and my colleagues discussed this between ourselves and decided that, since he was
not thriving in the supposed therapeutic environment of the hospital, his
wish should be respected. We realized it was a 'risky' discharge, but that
taking the risk was fully in accord with the Burford philosophy of care:
'...where the patient's experience and need for control in their lives is
recognized...'. Therefore Aaron was entitled to the opportunity to
succeed or fail at living at home within his limitations.

The hospital occupational therapist assessed his home resources and I
discussed Aaron's wishes with his GP so that he would be aware of my
rationale for facilitating Aaron's discharge. The GP's response, typically,
was laconic. 'If Aaron wishes that, then OK.'

I was not aware that I was asking the GP's permission for the discharge, and I am not sure if he interpreted it as such, but the use of 'OK'
would suggest that he did so. This raises the interesting point of sharing
one's work with other care workers who are not using the BNDU model.
Discussing patients' wishes with their GP, and conveying the doctor's
opinion to the patient, sometimes can be a useful way of relieving
anxiety. I suggested to one particular patient that she might benefit from
a weekend at home, but she would not consider it. I then discussed this
situation with her GP who agreed with me that it would appear to be
beneficial. When I told her that Dr Hilary approved she replied, 'Well, if
Dr Hilary thinks it is a good idea then it must be.'

With Aaron Maclean, however, his GP's opinion was marginal to our
decision to follow Aaron's wish. Aaron's home carer and the district
nurse were deeply sceptical, but as I wrote later in supervision notes:

> 'We felt we couldn't give any more care in hospital and he wouldn't let us near
> him...I offered him the choice to try it at home for the weekend – his morale
> was boosted – he wanted to try...He went home – he stayed bed bound, didn't
> eat or drink. He was seen by Ann [the district nurse] – she was distressed and
> angry at seeing him like that. She contacted me and fedback that sending him
> home was the wrong decision and that he should come back in. I agreed to this
> and explained that at the time I felt Aaron would benefit from the weekend to
> see for himself. Since he's been back he's been worse – he hasn't reflected at
> all on his visit home ... when prompted he just changed the subject.
>
> My feelings were that Ann was reacting as much to her work-load stress and
> blaming me for an inadequate discharge. She also remarked in this vein to
> others. I felt that her off-loading her stress clouded the issues for the patient. I
> asserted my right to have my decision accepted and the validity of my view-
> point.'

Reflection on the conflict of values

This experience illustrates the potentially problematic position of adopting a holistic philosophy of caring and having to communicate decisions based on that model to colleagues who either do not share or do not fully understand the meaning of the philosophy. The fundamental tension within this experience is the conflict of values in how I and the district nurse viewed the patient's experience and ways of working with the patient.

There are at least three questions resulting from this experience which need to be posed. Firstly, what does one do about dealing with conflicting values? The issue is raised within Burford's philosophy in that:

> 'Care ... is best given by those who care and have respect for each other within our respective accountable roles, despite differences of opinions at times, and who can share their feelings at appropriate times openly, and who mutually support others where needed...'
> (Johns 1992, p.89)

These words are chosen carefully to reflect the significance of the therapeutic team and allude to the difficulty which nurses have in being open to seeking and receiving valid feedback rather than falling back onto 'the harmonious team'. My experiences as a primary nurse at Burford support Johns' (1992) findings which suggest that assertiveness, facing conflict and sharing feelings are essential to the development of the therapeutic team. The countervailing culture of the harmonious team remains strongly resistant, like prevailing headwinds against which a cyclist might have to struggle.

A second related question concerns everyday ethics and 'technical ethics'. Seedhouse (1991) distinguishes between everyday ethics as a 'more intuitive and spontaneous reaction to life situations and dilemmas' and technical ethics as 'those more grounded in abstract theory and principles, and formed according to logic and analytic consistency.'

On an everyday level, I make judgements and decisions in my practice based on the juxtaposition of my own, my colleagues, and my patients' cultural, spiritual and personal beliefs in relation to emerging situations. I believe such an approach is acceptable, if not essential, for making our own decisions and taking action. The difficulty with my experience with the district nurse in discussing rationally our conflict over Aaron's care arose from our failure to make time to discuss and acknowledge everyday beliefs in context of the specific technical ethics that should have clearly influenced such a debate.

Thirdly, I wondered how the district nurse and I might have become comfortable with each other's point of view. My supervisor suggested that I ought to be assertive in telling her that I valued her contribution as part of the therapeutic team, that I recognized we had a problem of conflicting values, and that it was essential to discuss it openly. The difficulties we had experienced illustrate how painful it was, and as a consequence how defensive we were, to include each other fully in our therapeutic team.

Focusing on the patient

In attempting to reach Aaron Maclean, I reflected that he was a man with many barriers. I asked myself if I could see beyond the 'barriers'. What did I mean by this? I felt that whenever I tried to offer him any care and to work with him he responded mainly by blocking my approaches. Even when he did not physically turn away from me, he put up metaphorical barriers which stopped me getting any closer.

One morning I tried to spend the whole morning with him in an attempt to find a way out of his situation. He told me that he wanted to live, and I gave him feedback that he was killing himself by not eating and drinking. I noted that it was the first time with me that he had answered direct questions with direct answers. That seemed like a slice of progress and so I decided that rather than let care 'drift along', as it seemed to be doing, I had to continue to challenge him. In supervision I said:

> 'On reflection I feel very frustrated – I feel I achieved very little by challenging him ... this was not helped by interruptions – the telephone ringing, helping others. I had said to the others [staff] I wanted to concentrate on Aaron that morning – the other staff agreed to this. I was interrupted at important moments. I could have asserted my right to stay with him rather than respond to interruptions. I learnt how difficult this type of work is...'

I used the model of structured reflection (Johns 1993) to order my thoughts on this intervention, which helped me to understand myself better. I recognized that I wanted to '... widen the options of care and give nursing staff indication that something was being done'. It also brought my feelings into sharper and painful focus:

> 'I feel very sad and dissatisfied that I couldn't reach Aaron and feel that I didn't do all I could, but I don't know if it would have altered the situation ... when it was happening I felt powerless and at a loss – I didn't like it at all – it made me feel like a bad nurse, not a good primary nurse.'

Reading through this structured reflection with my supervisor after Aaron had died helped me to clarify further. The following conversation occurred between myself (the primary nurse (PN)) and my supervisor (S):

PN	When I confronted Aaron with the consequences of his actions he either clammed up or talked about something else...

S	What did you infer from that?

PN	The impression I got was that he was very afraid of what was happening to him – of losing control and dying. He couldn't admit it to me – I challenged him with the contradiction, but he didn't respond.

S	Perhaps you are getting too close?

PN	I feel I ought to have known what to do.

S	That sounds like the medical model.

PN	It does in a way – I didn't see it that way at the time – I just wanted to help him but I couldn't.

Summary of 'Case study – Aaron Maclean: a puzzle unsolved'

I began Aaron's case study with the statement that the holistic model for nursing practice is not a guarantee in itself that desired outcomes will be attained, but I feel that this in no way invalidates the model. Rather it suggests to me that the model is a powerful motivation for the practitioner to persist with rather than be wholly discouraged by difficult or problematic situations. Additionally, my experience with Aaron suggests that it would have been even more painful without the challenge, support and valid feedback of clinical supervision.

Postscript to 'Case study – Aaron Maclean: a puzzle unsolved'

I left the supervision session, during which I had reflected with deep anguish on Aaron's care, feeling that it was still problematic and that I felt very unhappy about it. I did not feel that 30 or 40 minutes talking had made it go away although I recognized supervision as an essential opportunity to talk confidentially about painful feelings.

At the time, I didn't believe it had helped much. But, cycling home along country roads to Witney, I felt a little better. The next morning, the first day of my substantial holiday in the six-and-a-half months since becoming a primary nurse at Burford, I woke up feeling much happier and reckoned that the reflections had enabled me to come to terms with myself within this experience.

In my next supervision session I said:

'Next morning I woke up and felt a "great weight" had lifted from me –

that I hadn't mucked up, and had been harder on myself than I needed to have been. It was like a delayed benefit from the session.'

Reflections on how using the BNDU model compares with using other models in previous experience

A year after I began using the BNDU model I feel as if I am still only scratching the surface of its potential. But compared with my previous application of nursing models I retain my first excitement and intuition that there *is* further potential in me to achieve my beliefs about nursing in practice. What do I mean by this?

Simply that there is something underneath the superficial structure of the model. It seems to have the potential to open the way to dealing with psycho-social aspects of care in a profound way. Sometimes I feel as if I have never listened to my patients before, and I hear such a wealth of information and insights that I cannot set it all down. Yet, what may appear to be a chance or passing remark provides us with invaluable insights into people's lives, how they are feeling and how they view themselves now and regarding the future.

Previously I have used the familiar, safe and bland cues of the Roper, Logan and Tierney model, with the activities of living and the life span continuum. When I wish to define specific physical activities, such as a mobility programme or care of a wound, this model would be adequate although limiting. Most practitioners will prescribe actions or interventions with which they are familiar already.

The BNDU model, by contrast, lends itself to widening out the possibilities. For example, in approaching the care of an extremely anxious man I outlined what he had told me, describing the ways I had observed his anxiety, and asked my colleagues to do likewise, to:

'... consider the strategies which might help [this person] to allay his anxieties, and, from interactions, note strategies which appear helpful or unhelpful.'

I am prepared to admit that I do not know all the approaches which might be therapeutic, and I see my colleagues, my patients and their carers as collaborators with me rather than slaves to my care plan or passive objects of care. It is clear that as a primary nurse I am responsible for initiating plans of care for my patients, but if either patients, carers or colleagues at any time find these inappropriate or inadequate, they are entitled to challenge or alter my plan provided they can offer a valid rationale.

Accountability relates to our belief at Burford that a primary nurse needs to grasp and explore the personal boundaries of autonomy, that is:

'... the freedom to make decisions within the boundaries of defined practice together with the freedom to act on those decisions.' (Johns 1990, p.886)

At Burford, this autonomy is balanced by collaboration:

'... of a therapeutic team that actively encourages and supports its members to explore and share their work.' (Johns 1990, p.889)

These are attractive words, but in reality it is extremely difficult to achieve because as qualified nurses we are acculturated to the harmonious team, which sees conflict and the giving and receiving of valid but uncomfortable feedback as too painful.

I find it easier to avoid conflict, but I also know that such evasion often prevents or delays outcomes which my patients, colleagues and I see as desirable. Avoidance does not permit resolution of conflict, but suppresses and fuels it. The outcomes of care within the framework of the BNDU model can be measured within the 'safe' forum of a group developing and critically examining standards of care to:

'... publicly demonstrate that the actions of nurses make a qualitative difference to people's lives.' (Johns 1991, p.1095)

However, it is in the field of day-to-day relationships with colleagues that escaping from the old ideas is hard, and the application of new ones equally so. In other environments of care, I have felt constrained by a rigid vertical hierarchy, and an uneasy combination of a biological systems model within a dominant medical model. Psychological care was largely unplanned or defined superficially in modes such as, 'Give the patient time to ask questions and express anxieties' or the ubiquitous, 'Give reassurance'. Patients' profound psychological and spiritual needs were addressed at times, but I suspect this was despite the nursing model not because of it.

'The Burford model has emerged out of practice ... and returns to practice for testing and increasing sophistication.' (Johns 1991, p.1097)

Through the cue questions and the use of Special Intervention sheets I am able to explore my caring potential and achieve patient-centred therapeutic care. It is in my hands as a clinical practitioner. Now, with some of my patients, I note that most of my care planning develops through the Special Intervention sheets as I recognize the centrality of their psycho-social and spiritual needs.

My attention to the BNDU model has been a long adventurous journey – an odyssey. My understanding of and value for the model has deepened during this continuous journey. Evaluation of the model is an area which requires further reflection – as with other accounts in this book.

Through the use of case studies I have attempted to show something of the nature of my personal journey in tandem with my patients and colleagues. I have tried to highlight how the BNDU model provides me with a challenging and dynamic framework in tune with my beliefs as a nurse, for the benefit of my patients and my colleagues.

It is of particular pertinence as I write because we are preparing for a critical review of the philosophy for practice, an event I am eagerly anticipating. It seems a paradox that I feel attuned to the model, and the model fits the practice to which I aspire, but I do not feel attuned to the philosophy. This is not because I have profound disagreements with it, but I recognize how:

'A philosophy for practice offers tangible vision that becomes a foundation for change.' (Johns 1991, p.1097)

and I welcome the opportunities my practice offers for change.

I began this chapter with a quotation from Oliver Sacks and I close it with another (1990, p.xix):

'In the study of our most complex sufferings and disorder of being we are compelled to scrutinise the deepest, darkest, and most fearful parts of ourselves, the parts we all strive to deny or not see. The thoughts which are most difficult to grasp or express are those which touch on this forbidden region and re-awaken in us our strongest denials and our most profound intuitions.'

References

Johns, C.C. (1990) Autonomy of primary nurses: the need to both facilitate and limit autonomy in practice. *Journal of Advanced Nursing*, **15**, 886–94.

Johns, C.C. (1991) The Burford Nursing Development Unit holistic model of nursing practice. *Journal of Advanced Nursing*, **16**, 1090–98.

Johns, C.C. (1992) Ownership and the harmonious team: barriers to developing the therapeutic nursing team in primary nursing. *Journal of Clinical Nursing,* **1,** 89–94.

Johns, C.C. (1993) Profession supervision. *Journal of Nursing Management,* **1**(1), 9–18.

Johnson, D.E. (1974) Development of theory; a requisite for nursing as a primary health profession. *Nursing Research,* **23**(5), 373–7.

Sacks, O. (1990) Awakenings, (revised ed). Picador, London.

Schon, D.A. (1983) *The Reflective Practitioner: How Professionals Think in Action.* Basic Books, New York.

Seedhouse, D. (1991) *Ethics The Heart of Health Care.* John Wiley, Chichester.

Street, A.F. (1992) *Inside Nursing: A Critical Ethnography of Clinical Nursing Practice.* State University of New York Press, New York.

Editor's commentary

Within the case study of Madge Brown, Roger Cowell illustrates how he came to confront himself and subsequently his colleagues with the failure to see Madge as a person and to consider the perceptions of 'who a patient is'. In recognizing Madge's feelings of dehumanisation, her lack of self-esteem was realised and Roger's positive intervention led to mutually satisfying experiences for Madge, himself and his colleagues. Satisfaction is an important element in maintaining a sense of commitment to caring and Roger expressed his commitment to Madge and her husband Bill by following up aspects of care after Madge had been discharged.

Arranging this discharge created conflict with the district nurse and highlights the potential difficulty of using the model in association with others who do not share similar philosophies. Many nurses have not had the opportunity to express themselves and embrace the meaning of caring in practice. Roger himself felt that prior to Burford his own beliefs about caring had been squashed in oppressive hierarchical and medically dominated systems.

Another aspect highlighted in this chapter is the limitations of written communication in ensuring effective continuity of care. This difficulty with written communication as a means of passing on what practitioners want to say and for ensuring continuity of care is apparent and seems to reflect the oral tradition within nursing (Street 1992) and the essential intuitive nature of emotional aspects of care. Understanding these issues led to the development of Special Intervention sheets at Burford as a more expressive and meaningful way to communicate psychological and social aspects of patient care.

This chapter also demonstrates with the second case study (concerning Johny Arthur) how using the BNDU model leads to writing about a patient in a narrative style that is a reflection of seeing the person in a holistic sense. This style also applies to assessments and nursing notes as recorded on Special Intervention sheets. This focus on holistic communication and the making explicit of personal feelings is clearly better than following an hierarchical approach to communication as apparent with the usual nursing process.

In this second case study Roger portrays his commitment to the patient through his advocacy of this vulnerable person entering a long stay care institution. His intention is to help others understand this man.

In the third case study (concerning Aaron Maclean), Roger considers his own anxieties about the reflective nature of the BNDU model fuelling self-doubt and not 'allowing' him to escape from anxiety through rationalizing the situation. In doing so, the need for organizational support systems to sustain his therapeutic work is demonstrated. Reflection in group supervision illustrated that support from colleagues was more espoused than a reality in practice at this time.

In striving to make sense of his feelings of responsibility towards Aaron and the conflict between himself and the district nurse over Aaron's discharge home, the ethical and involvement dimensions of therapeutic work are highlighted. Commitment to patients always has a risk of leading to involvement where the practitioner's emotions become entwined with those of the patient causing distorted thinking and personal anxiety – in Aaron's case illustrated by Roger 'blaming' himself.

His reflection on using the BNDU model in his practice indicates how sensitive he has become towards his patients and towards his colleagues, although not always with desirable outcomes. As Roger emphasizes, the development of the therapeutic team to mutually support each other on a day-to-day basis has been difficult to achieve because of the resilience of the embedded culture of the harmonious team.

This chapter also draws attention to the consequences of nurses' efforts to make philosophies based on human caring a reality in practice. Pursuing the cue questions leads inexorably to engagement with patients and confrontation of the nurse with the perception of 'who a nurse is'. Roger makes a number of references to his work in 'supervision', and how supervision, through guiding his learning through shared reflective experiences, enables him to make sense of some of these issues.

Of course, reflective practice and using a reflective model of practice are two dimensions of being a reflective practitioner – and hence complement each other. The BNDU cue questions are a device for Roger to reflect-in-action, immediately and simultaneously being tuned into himself, the philosophy for practice and the patient or relative.

Planning care is not so much a linear process as encouraged within the nursing process, but the aesthetic grasping, interpreting, envisioning and responding appropriately within the situation as outlined in Chapter 2. The model enables creative expression of the self rather like painting a picture or writing a poem – it gives meaning to the expression 'the art of nursing'.

Chapter 5

Just Following Care? Reflections of Associate Nurses in Using the BNDU Model at Burford

Kate Butcher and Jan Dewing

In this chapter we reflect on our use of the BNDU model from the perspectives of our associate nurse roles at Burford. This account reflects our personal involvement in practice and using the model. As such, we write in the first person. Webb (1992) states that it is acceptable to write in the first person when one has played a crucial role in shaping the formation or the ideas being presented. Writing in the first person enables us to assert to readers that our shared reflections on the use of the BNDU model in practice are personal.

The role of the associate nurse

Our roles, as associate nurses are very different. One of us, Kate, is employed as an associate nurse, whilst the other, Jan, works as an associate nurse within her contracted role as lecturer/practitioner and hospital manager. We therefore bring different perspectives, knowledge and skills to our mutual roles.

The role of the associate nurse is essentially to carry out the prescribed care planned by the primary nurse and to respond to changing circumstances in the absence of the primary nurse as appropriate (Manthey 1980). In fulfilling this role, the BNDU model gives us 'artistic licence', in a positive sense, to be the nurses we are, and to strive to become the nurses we hope to become. In other words, we are practitioners in our own right, with beliefs and feelings that are important determinants in the care we give.

From the perspective of a lecturer/practitioner my clinical work can either be given over several spans of duty so I can practise nursing for myself or as a role model for other staff or it may be an occasional span 'here and there'. I need to be able to nurse in a clinical role for myself because I am a nurse. I need to have relationships with patients, relatives, nurses and other clinical staff because it provides a source of motivation and questioning for me to carry out the other aspects of my role in education and management.

In the latter instance, working 'here and there' would tend to be where I was asked to work as an associate nurse, at short notice perhaps because of sickness. In both instances my practice tends to be intense. Because I know I am working with patients and my colleagues for a fixed period of time I want to work as effectively as I can to maximize my contribution to patient care.

I would argue that in both instances, but especially the latter one, use of the model, particularly by the primary nurses, enables me to gain a greater insight into the patients and their care. This is especially so when working for one span of duty. I know that the hand-over of care I receive, the care plans and other forms of communication tell me about the patient and have not been mentally processed through a collection of nursing frameworks in which the patient's perspective can be lost. The Burford model enables me to gain a clear insight of the patient's perspective of the meaning of their illness, together with the feelings and ideas the primary nurses have about the patient's care.

On a very practical level this saves me much time in trying to re-establish the unwritten and often covert ground rules of relationships with patients. The obvious advantages are that it enables me to feel more part of the nursing team and that care for the patients has more continuity and consistency, even if it is being delivered by a 'part-time nurse'.

From the perspective of other associate nurses, who may be part-time workers or newly qualified nurses (as one of us is), or nurses returning to work following a break in their careers, using the model may prove to be more challenging. Many of these associate nurses may be lacking in their professional or personal confidence. To get the best out of the model requires nurses to be creative and this often means taking risks. Taking risks exposes the nurses to their patients and colleagues and perhaps this requires great personal and professional confidence.

Personal philosophies

The starting point to working creatively with the Burford model of nursing is to examine one's own philosophy of nursing. We both share many similarities in our personal philosophies of nursing, yet in many ways they are very different. That our philosophies share many similarities is reassuring; this is necessary in order to offer patients consistent and congruent care (Johns 1991). We do not feel our personal philosophies have to be exactly the same and they are not. Perhaps the main reason they are different is that they are never complete and hence are at different stages in their conception and construction as would be expected with our different nursing careers to date.

Developing a personal philosophy of nursing practice is a continuous process. For us it involves reflecting on our experiences with practice and 'fitting' them with our own values and beliefs and accumulated knowledge. This reflection often highlights contradictions between our beliefs and values and the way we practice which require further reflection to reduce.

Our personal philosophies are reflected in the hospital philosophy of practice. The Burford model of nursing, because it is developed from our collective beliefs and values, reflects our personal philosophies of nursing, the way we think and the way in which we practise nursing. As Johnston (1989) states, conceptual models represent their author's view of nursing. Many authors would claim this to be true with all conceptual models of nursing. We have not been able to share in the philosophies of other nursing models and, as such, they lack personal meaning for us.

Kate's experiences

The following case studies aim to demonstrate to the reader the use of the BNDU model in practice and each study highlights a different aspect. All have had particular relevance in my development as a nurse, that is, they have all been valuable learning experiences. Each has been discussed in my supervision sessions to enable further learning, and thus I am able to present them as logical and ordered scenarios.

Case study – Jack and Sarah

This first case study uses the situation of the associate nurse progressing from working alongside the primary nurse to becoming the actual primary nurse for an individual due to the resignation of the primary nurse. At this point I had been qualified as a registered nurse for only eight weeks.

Jack Roberts was admitted to Burford, accompanied by his wife Sarah, following a collapse in his garden. He was a retired naval officer, 'a gentleman' as his GP described him, but now he was aphasic with a dense right-sided weakness. Sarah was distraught especially due to the fact that they had only married two years previously.

Along with care planning for Jack's rehabilitation following his diagnosed Cerebral Vascular Accident, care was also offered to Sarah. This is common at Burford due to our assessment question 'Who is this person?' To answer this question fully necessitates a holistic assessment which naturally extends to the family. Since Sarah was also Jack's support in life – this is linked with the cue question 'What support does this person have in life?' – it was natural that Sarah's needs were also considered. A Special Intervention sheet was developed headed 'Counselling Mrs Roberts', upon which were recorded relevant comments and conversations from Sarah which indicated her level of coping with Jack's condition.

The primary nurse had spoken with Sarah on several occasions so when I took responsibility for Jack's care I found the recorded notes of considerable value. Comments such as:

'It's a complete reversal of roles. Jack was always the strong partner.'

and

'It's the lack of communication I can't deal with; we used to talk so much...'

were recorded along with information such as the fact that Sarah felt that Jack should be discharged to a nursing home rather than to their home on the completion of his care at Burford. She also explained how difficult she found helping Jack to wash and dress despite wanting to help. Such recorded information helped me to validate her actions such as unexpected hesitancy and shyness when I became responsible for their care.

This case study illustrates the holism of the BNDU model in that care was extended to the family of the individual, in my experience an often neglected issue of care as partners are seen as individuals in their own right, but less often as an integral part of the individual requiring care. Sarah and Jack were a couple very much involved in each other's lives. Therefore to care for Jack we had to care for Sarah. This meant that we had to offer Sarah some of the care that she would have expected from Jack had he been able to give it, for example, emotional support since Jack could not talk.

This experience highlighted the value of the cue question 'How do they view the future for themselves and others?' Since Jack could not tell us we had to ask Sarah, and it was then that we discovered not only

Sarah's wish for nursing home accommodation for Jack but also all the stress she was experiencing which we could help to alleviate. Since the cue questions are precisely that, a cue, a prompt to aid thinking, each cue question does not require an answer, but the ones highlighted in this study proved themselves to be invaluable when planning care for Jack. Without these I imagine that care offered to Sarah would have been inconsistent between different staff members, and that Jack's future may not have been considered with as much individualization as it was.

The use of the model eased the transition of my role from associate nurse to primary nurse for this family in that all the information I initially needed was provided through the assessment and care plans. I had only to make myself better known to all those involved and adapt to the altered responsibility. Thanks to the BNDU model I felt I had already begun to 'know' the family and therefore felt that the care I could offer would be individualized. I had never before felt this when reading notes which had been written based on another model. However, had my practical experience been greater I may have been able to enhance the care we offered to Sarah, rather than merely following the plan already set.

The model allows for a considerable amount of creativity on the part of each nurse involved in its use, but to achieve this, experience and confidence are necessary. I do not feel that we offered a poor standard of care to Jack and Sarah, but acknowledge through reflection that we may have improved the care. The extent to which I was able to be therapeutic with Jack and Sarah depended very much at the time on my degree of experience, and I felt quite strongly at this point that a nurse with greater experience than myself may have worked differently (low self-esteem eight weeks after qualifying as a nurse placed a voice in my head saying 'better', rather than 'differently').

However, the BNDU model focuses on each nurse's areas for development due to its reflective nature, and thus turns each experience into a learning situation. Therefore, although I had some negative feelings I still felt supported by the model since I felt that any nurse, regardless of amount of experience, would have learnt something and so I was not alone!

Case study – Mildred

This second case study illustrates my changed role to a 'trainee' primary nurse, that is, acting as primary nurse to one patient with support from other staff members. This gives the opportunity to practise the skills of a primary nurse whilst having the support of other staff members who recognize the 'novice' state.

Mildred Baker was admitted for rehabilitation following a fall on ice when she sustained fractures of the humerus and tibia. She also had multiple chronic health problems to deal with, for example, polymyalgia and diverticulitis. She had a close and loving family who visited regularly, and a strong religious faith, both of which provided her with support for life.

I wrote in my assessment of Mildred that she '... relies heavily on the fact that she can be of help to others and consequently feels useless' (at being in hospital unable to physically help herself, never mind others), and that, 'she feels she no longer has her health' due to the fractures; chronic conditions were quite obviously incorporated into an already adjusted concept of health, but now Mildred had to temporarily adjust her concept again. These comments acknowledged, and maybe even predicted, Mildred's lack of coping mechanisms to deal with such a situation and therefore allowed me to plan for such.

Three weeks later when writing on her continuous assessment sheet I wrote:

'Although her physiotherapy is progressing well, Mildred does not seem to believe in this, or have the faith in herself, relying more and more on our reassurance.'

Continuing assessment of the individual is demanded by the BNDU model as we develop a greater understanding of the person and develop trusting relationships enabling deeper insight into their situation, and because a person's state of health often fluctuates, as in the case of Mildred. As primary nurse, I was responsible for assessing Mildred and I found the cue questions of great use, especially with regard to psychosocial care – the questions 'Who is this person?' and 'What support does this person have in life?' being the most relevant to Mildred.

However, writing care plans to deal with the identified problems was not easy as whatever I wrote seemed to patronize and be stereotyped, for example:

Mildred is anxious due to hospital admission.
Goal: To reassure.
Actions: Give Mildred time to talk about her feelings.

Such documentation made me feel as though the care I would then be giving was not individualized because I had written it so many times previously as a student, and read it so many times too. To overcome this feeling I found that it was useful to use the Special Intervention sheets, relating them to her increased dependence for support upon the staff rather than her gaining this from her family or faith as she had done on admission.

I wrote how I thought staff should approach Mildred, but rather than being prescriptive in my manner, rather than writing 'If Mildred says she feels useless tell her that you understand but that this isn't the case,' I was suggestive as I believed that the approaches of other staff could be equally valid. This was important to me as I have felt as a student that I was only performing a set of functions that someone else thought appropriate and that my individuality and thoughts could not show through the care. This attitude made me feel de-valued as a nurse and I did not wish to make my colleagues feel this way in their care of Mildred.

Special Intervention sheets demand a creativity from the practitioner as they are actually a blank sheet of paper. This can be both empowering and stressful. The empowerment arises from the acknowledgement of the nurse's skill at developing individualized care, the freedom to be creative within collective beliefs, and the chance to work as a team in fulfilling the challenge set out by the sheets. However, stress can quickly arise from this freedom, the stress of 'not knowing' the best action to take because the situation has not been encountered previously by the nurse, of feeling inexperienced and incompetent.

This latter point is also highlighted through the freedom of the assessment tool. Whereas for example, Roper *et al.*'s model (used as a comparison because this was encountered on each ward I worked on as a student) would expect some consideration of the physical aspects of care such as elimination or breathing, the Burford model asks the vague question (as I interpreted it since it did not direct me to think of specific activities of living), 'what health event brings this person into hospital?' For a recently qualified practitioner as I was at the time (approximately four months) this did not guide me to think about problems such as constipation due to diverticulitis.

Whilst I acknowledge that the reason behind such an omission was my own inexperience, the model was not the guide I had hoped for, therefore making the situation more stressful. Whilst I am not suggesting that other models excuse practitioners from thinking for themselves, they may direct or focus the thought more quickly thus seeming less stressful at the time. On reflection I would now suggest that the more directive models could be seen as being restrictive if not used to their full potential, for example Roper *et al.*'s model is often interpreted as only being a list of twelve activities of daily living, and I suggest that the BNDU model is liberating in its use.

I found the cue question 'How does this person make me feel?' to be of incredible value during Mildred's stay as I found my relationship with her changing throughout her admission. I discussed the situation in my supervision.

> As Mildred gets to know me better I feel that she is manipulating me.

In terms of being therapeutic, having access to such feelings was invaluable since I was able to recognize the reasoning behind my actions, for example, becoming more detached from Mildred, and through reflection I was able to identify the effects upon Mildred of this withdrawal and also predict how I could cope with my feelings more effectively.

The model, being reflective in nature by asking 'How does this person make me feel?', put me in contact with my own feelings more than I had ever been and so enabled me to act positively to overcome negative feelings such as the manipulation. This was a large issue for me in caring for Mildred as I felt that we were moving away from working in a partnership with one another to Mildred being 'in charge'. This seems paradoxical: my aim was ultimately for Mildred to be in control of her situation, but through her manner she was not making informed choices and therefore I felt I was battling against her. Had we remained in the 'partnership' state I could have offered advice more comfortably and so prevented some of my stress.

This case study has identified a weakness in the BNDU model for student/newly qualified staff: not providing enough structure in some cases for the optimum level of care planning. It has also highlighted a positive stressor – that of creativity – and the value of some of the cue questions.

Case study – Bert

In this description of Bert's admission to Burford I assumed the most commonly portrayed role of the associate nurse, that of following the care as planned by the primary nurse and reporting any changes needed for their approval (Pearson 1988; Manthey 1973).

Bert Johnson was an intelligent and articulate man, widely travelled and very knowledgeable. He was admitted to Burford for respite care on a regular basis as he had worsening emphysema and was reliant on oxygen therapy. He was interested in the concept of individualized care and assisted the primary nurse in the development of his care plan. During the admission upon which this case study is based, Bert identified the problem 'I feel unable to spend my days in Burford as I would at home', with the underlying current of now being unable to live his life as he used to due to the emphysema restricting his activities.

During each previous admission Bert seemed to enjoy making staff feel uncomfortable by almost humiliating them due to their lack of knowledge, for example, he would order his lunch in Dutch. Due to this habit staff would try to have minimal contact with him due to the unpleasant feelings he created within them. For this reason there were areas of his assessment not completed as comprehensively as they could have been.

Bert Johnson's admission occurred during a quiet period at work. Therefore I decided to get to know Bert on a less superficial level, to dispel the preconceptions I had gathered from other staff. I did this ostensibly for my own reasons – Bert made me feel uncomfortable and I wanted to put an end to this. Whenever I had free time I would sit with Bert, allowing him to lead the conversations. I found that by giving him some of my attention and time when he knew I could be relaxing he became less demanding and critical, grateful for honesty from the staff, for example, 'This is interesting but can we continue it later when I have more time to spend with you?' He also became more honest himself, speaking of his feelings and anxieties relating to his deteriorating condition.

I spoke with the primary nurse and discussed my 'breakthrough' and wrote a Special Intervention sheet for the benefit of all staff:

> On talking to Bert I have found him to be a pleasant, interesting and considerate man. He knows how he is perceived by others – 'a moaner', 'demanding', 'boring', 'a miserable old man' – but also expresses feelings of loneliness and a fear of his deteriorating condition and eventual death. I feel we have not been aware of this situation in the past and have therefore treated Bert a little brusquely.
>
> I therefore challenge staff's attitudes towards Bert (including my own) and suggest that we do spend time with him when we can. He does understand that we have other people to care for too, and only expects politeness and honesty.

The prompts for me writing about my experience in this way were the cue questions 'Who is this person?' and 'How does this person make me feel?' which lead to the answering of the questions 'How is this person feeling?' and 'What is important for this person to make their stay in hospital more comfortable?' Whilst these questions had been considered by the primary nurse, different answers were developed by both of us highlighting the subjective nature of the cue questions and hence the assessment of each individual. It also emphasizes the need for good relationships between team members.

The cue question 'How does this person make me feel?' allowed me to access my feelings and then deal with them, thus ensuring that I remained available to work therapeutically with Bert. This was of great importance to me as many other staff members had rejected him and I therefore saw a challenge in working with Bert. It also prevented me from rejecting him too.

Through 'simple' actions such as listening to Bert I was able to relate our behaviours to Berne's (1964) theory of Transactional Analysis. I identified in my supervision that Bert 'had been treating me like a child, humiliating me with his language', but that 'I had responded as an adult and that is where we had difficulties in communication'. According to Berne's theory, in any interaction we can adopt any one of three roles: parent, adult or child. Clear lines of communication exist between like roles or opposite roles, but problems occur, for example, between roles of parent and adult.

Once a relationship of honesty had been developed with Bert we were able to relate to one another either as adult to adult or as parent to child; (if Bert reverted to his 'humiliation tactics' I was able to respond positively by moving myself into the child role of accepting the parent's teaching, thus saving myself from humiliation and protecting Bert from receiving my anger should this have occurred.)

The key points from this case study relating to the model were:

- The interpretation of the cue questions, i.e. the subjective nature.
- The development of a therapeutic relationship (one where both Bert and myself received positive feelings).
- The notion of holism (Bert participating in care planning).
- The link between all the cue questions (one leading to another).
- The use of the Special Intervention sheet to enable all willing staff to develop a more positive relationship with Bert.

The model and a developing career

From these three case studies it can be seen how experience and confidence affect the use of the model. Whilst it was of value in the first study, as a newly qualified practitioner I did not have the confidence to expand upon it. Following the plans of the primary nurse was made easy due to the thoroughness of the assessment, but inexperience inhibited my developing it further. Possibly with a model such as Roper *et al.*'s the handing over of care would not have been as thorough, but I may have been able to plan further myself.

In the second case study it can be seen that confidence is growing and I am able to assess a patient reasonably well myself using the cue questions and Special Intervention sheets. However, the model inhibited me at that time from considering a more subtle area of physical care. Following another model may have provided me with inspiration for a better care plan for physical problems, but a poorer one for psycho-social ones.

The final description of care demonstrates much more confidence in the use of the model, to the point where I am able to consider my own influence upon an individual and vice versa, and thus the model leads to much more therapeutic care being given.

Jan's experiences

The following case study describes my admission assessment in the absence of the primary nurse. In many senses this was a 'holiday activity' by me in my role as an associate nurse, yet it provided much valuable information for the primary nurse who used it as a basis for developing her relationship with the patient rather than repeating the assessment.

Case study – Joan

Joan was a 67-year-old woman who came to the hospital for assessment following a request by her GP. The day before her admission she reported a sudden loss of function in her legs. There did not appear to be an apparent reason for this. The history given to the GP was unclear as both Joan and her family were very panicked by what was happening. Joan's sister and daughter had looked after her on the sofa overnight.

Very quickly, during talking with Joan, I could see that it was not appropriate to carry out a detailed assessment; Joan was very tired, she had had little sleep the night before and she was anxious about being in hospital. She got into bed with all her clothes on, even her coat, and declined to take them off for several hours.

Despite being very conscious of my interviewing skills and techniques, Joan gave very short factual responses to questions. She was unable to answer questions that were open ended and those that related to how she felt about what was happening. She sat very still in the bed and did not respond. Her eye contact with me, despite my seating and body positioning, was minimal.

During an initial assessment I am always pleased if I gain an insight into the person and their perception of their health. I regard assessments as an ongoing process, like a jigsaw, and think the initial assessment should be as non-invasive as possible. The model reflects this shared belief that assessment should be sensitive and non-invasive. For Joan it was not appropriate to continue with a detailed assessment. It was even possible that she did not want to talk at all. Following the interview I began to reflect on why I thought this way, using the cue questions below.

'How does this patient make me feel?'

I felt as if Joan was not interested in talking to me, but I was able to understand that this was not personal. Had I thought that, I might not have gone back to her or questioned myself any further about what was happening. I realized that I was reading her body language and her verbal and non-verbal cues which were indicating to me that she was not interested in talking.

However, it seemed to me that her face had a mask expression almost as if she was unresponsive or devoid of emotion or that her emotion was suppressed. Her voice was flat and expressionless. I began to consider that she may be like this because she was very frightened or that the loss of functioning had affected her non-verbal and verbal communication skills or that she was poorly skilled in communicating her feelings. I also considered that she may have another pathological problem which we did not know about, such as Parkinson's disease, or that she was taking medications that caused her to appear unreactive or devoid of emotion.

I had also noticed the way in which her family assisted her to settle into bed. I observed them relating to her almost as if she was a child. They talked to her using simple language with a lot of instructions and Joan did not always respond to them. Although I thought that their behaviour could be a reflection of their anxiety, it seemed to be deeper than this.

I needed to consider the next cue question.

'How can I best help this person?'

When I shared my feelings of uncertainty about not knowing how best to help Joan at this time because I could not work out what she wanted and because she did not seem able to communicate with me clearly, the daughter and sister immediately knew what I meant. They told me that it was an effect of the medication she was taking and that she could not help it. I asked them how they thought she was feeling. They told me things that Joan said and how she behaved when anxious. They said Joan needed lots of reassurance and lots of affection. They also said she did not seem to acknowledge it, but she did appreciate it. This then added another dimension to my assessment of Joan. It led me to ask the next cue question.

'How is this person feeling?'

After reflecting on this new information I was able to think that Joan might not be feeling as calm or detached as she had appeared. Her sister and daughter described to me how Joan switched off completely when she was worried about something. I knew now that she was not unreactive or devoid of emotion, but I had thought that she wanted to be left on her own, and wondered if she was unable to ask for help and was therefore feeling very isolated. Perhaps she had perceived my behaviour as showing little concern for her because I had not shown her affection.

From a distance I observed her resting in bed and her sleep pattern, such as her movements and her breathing. When I assessed that she was no longer asleep but lying with her eyes closed I went and sat beside her and quietly said, 'When you feel like opening your eyes I will help you to do what you want to do.' After a few minutes she opened her eyes and said 'I need to use the toilet, but I don't know if I can.' When she said this her face was still expressionless as was her voice.

I knew that for Joan it was becoming very frightening because she was losing her functions very quickly; it seemed to her that every time she tried to do something else she had lost the ability. She was perplexed and could not make sense of what was happening to her. She needed help, but felt cut off from other people because of the way she presented herself and the way other people interpreted their first impressions of her.

Because I stopped and reflected on the events surrounding Joan's admission using the cue questions flexibly I was able to see how the situation might be from Joan's perspective. This insight then influenced the direction and provision of nursing care I was able to give. It also influenced the information I gave to the nurse coming on for night duty.

Using the cue questions

The cue questions form an adaptable framework for practice. As Salvage (1990) states, nursing models can open up new channels of communication and provide a fresh focus of work interest for the benefit of nurses as well as patients. When primary nurses are handing over their patients to us, we know that they are using the information from the cue questions as a basis for their impressions of the patient. We are able to internalize their thoughts, ideas and information using the cue questions to guide us in forming our own internal framework. This can lead us to ask questions about the patient, the nurse–patient relationship or the nursing care that becomes focused around the cue questions.

During practice, information gained from experiences shared with patients, relatives and nurses can be added to existing knowledge about the patient within the framework. The cue questions seek to assist us with validating or further questioning our assumptions or interpretations, as the case study with Joan demonstrated. It is important to acknowledge that we do not automatically accept new information if it does not easily fit with the framework of cues. If this happens that it is necessary to question the validity of the framework. We recognize that the model is new and must be continually tested – both the theory in practice and the practice with the theory.

The cue questions can often act as stem questions. The acquisition of knowledge can lead to adapting or expanding the cue question.

For example, consider the cue question 'Who is this person?' At times it might not be possible to see who the person is as this involves an understanding of their past, their present and their future, but it may be appropriate to ask who is this person I see *now*. Seeing someone does not just involve the visual senses but all the senses including intuition. Joan's case is an example of not being fully able to see who this person was immediately after admission. However, it did not mean that the nurse could not assess the patient. This also demonstrates the versatility of the cues over time.

One of the main points to make is that during assessment or any type of work with patients the cue questions need never be spoken as they are written. With some patients it might be appropriate, but with most patients in our experience it has not been appropriate. The questions act as cues or stems on which to base assessment, nursing care and evaluation of care. We are free to work with patients using any strategies we have. When we collect and reflect on the information gained we then use the cue questions to form a framework.

Case study – Dorothy

The following information could be a standard nursing entry in the nursing notes following a span of duty. The patient is a woman of 97 years of age. She has been admitted for treatment of an infection. During her admission she was confused and expressed paranoid ideas. She declared she wanted to be left to die. The GP documented that her wishes should be respected. The nurse wrote:

> This patient has been very demanding and difficult. She has been aggressive to the staff. She is confused and disorientated. She has constantly been shouting and swearing. She has refused any care and refused all fluids.

This entry is reflective of a de-personalized approach by the nurse. The patient has no name. She is described as being demanding and difficult by the nurse because she does not accept the care that is on offer. The nurse is not able to form a relationship with the patient and cannot use any helpful strategies, so rather than identify this weakness in her practice the nurse projects her discomfort onto the patient.

The nurse justifies her inability to care for the patient by saying the patient is confused and disorientated. These two terms are often used together and inappropriately by nurses. Because it is assumed that this patient is not to be actively treated, the nurse does not question the doctor's assessment of the patient's wishes and accordingly ascribes a low priority to trying to work therapeutically with the patient.

The same entry written following using the cue questions as a framework might look something like this:

> Dorothy has been distressed this morning. She is not as disorientated as she was last night. She appears confused. She makes reference to God punishing her by sending thunder and lightning. However, I feel that from Dorothy's perspective this makes sense. The lightning was the bright morning sun shining on her face. The tree obscured the sun intermittently and it suddenly hit her in the eyes. In view of her poor vision the effect of the light seems like lightning. The thunder is probably the main door opening and closing. Her comments about the thunder correlate with someone opening and closing the door. I have attended to these things and Dorothy is not so distressed.
>
> Dorothy continues to believe I am trying to poison her and strikes out if I offer her any water. She is very thirsty and states she is dying for a drink but cannot take it. I have arranged for her friends to bring in water and her favourite foods and see if she will take it from them. I have found that the most useful way to help Dorothy is to spend a few minutes with her and then she will take sips of water. If I spend more than a few minutes she becomes distressed and agitated by my presence and refuses water.
>
> I am trying to find ways of getting her to eat and drink. But I am finding it very frustrating. I believe she wants to drink, but thinks she is being poisoned. I do not believe that Dorothy is ready to die. I feel she has a mental health problem which prevents her from helping herself. It is this that I find the most difficult as it is blocking Dorothy from accepting our help.

This case study demonstrates several key points:

(1) It shows the nurse attempting to see the situation from the patient's perspective by trying to understand the thunder and lightning.

(2) It shows use of several cues. These include considering how the patient might be feeling, how the nurse can best help the patient and how the patient is making the nurse feel.

(3) The helping strategies the nurse is trying to work out are small ones, such as ways to get Dorothy to drink. But it shows that this is still important as it is often the smaller aspects of caring for patients that get left out from nursing records and nursing discussions.

(4)   It shows that it is important that these aspects of care are acknowledged so that they can be learnt by other nurses.

(5)   It shows that the nurse recognizes the need to make positive use of the support Dorothy has from her friends.

(6)   It shows that the nurse is considering how the patient is affecting her and how she feels about her care and about the patient. This nurse recognizes that she feels frustrated by not being able to help Dorothy in the way she intends to, but does not blame Dorothy for that or try and cover up her inability to help Dorothy.

Case study – Bob

The following conversation occurred between myself (the associate nurse (AN)) and Bob (a patient) after helping him in the toilet. Following his lunch he had been incontinent of faeces and had needed to be cleaned and have his clothing changed.

Bob   Are you the cook?

AN   No. Is there something you would like to tell the cook?

Bob   No.

(Pause)

AN   Do you think the cook would be doing what I just have done?

Bob   Who are you then – a nurse?

AN   Yes – is that a surprise?

Bob   God save us! Why don't you do your job properly?

AN   What should I have done? Please tell me.

Bob   What you're paid for. Standing around doing nothing. Worse than useless. You should be helping me rather than making me do things.

AN   So what have I done? What was undressing you, washing you, dressing you and helping you to walk back here meant to be?

Bob   If you can call that help.

AN   How would you like us to help you?

Bob   Do your job properly. Are you satisfied with what you do? You make a poor nurse.

AN   I am finding it difficult to know how to help you because you're not treating me as an equal. We can only help you if you let us. You have to want us to help you.

Bob   It seems to me you keep everyone alive as long as you can so they suffer and you do as little as you can.

AN   I can understand it might seem like that to you. Many of the patients here, although they are disabled and unwell, may not feel like you ... Do you feel you are suffering?

Bob   If you are going to lecture me you can clear off...

Prior to this conversation Bob had never entered into a dialogue with any of the nurses. We had the feeling he was angry about having a stroke and he resented the way it had disabled him. We also felt that he did not value what the nurses were trying to do with him. He dismissed our care and yet declined to enter into any partnership to work out something better for himself. He even declined to negotiate partnership of any kind with his primary nurse.

In this conversation these views are confirmed. By reflecting-in-action I recognized that I had the opportunity to establish a dialogue with Bob because of the way in which he spoke and the preceding events. I tried to work out, as the conversation progressed, what Bob was feeling, how I could best find out more about who this person was and how I could best help him. I recognized that Bob was trying to devalue both me and my help because he felt angry with himself for needing the help. I had to get beyond this in order to achieve a therapeutic interaction with him. I also let Bob see that the nurses wanted to work with him, confirming and supporting the work being done by his primary nurse. It would have been very easy to have risen to the insults Bob gave out.

Although Bob ended the conversation when it became too close to him, some valuable insights into how Bob was feeling about himself and how he felt about his future and his nursing care were made. I also felt it was appropriate for Bob to end the conversation in his way so that he felt he still had some control over the situation.

On reflection I can identify ways in which I could have tried to facilitate the conversation to develop further, so I realize that this is not a 'textbook' example of communication skills, but it is important to provide real examples of what happens and how the model is used as a dynamic framework in practice.

Use of Special Intervention sheets

The use of Special Intervention sheets enables nurses to be creative. They can be used in many ways to increase nurses' awareness about aspects of care that are difficult to factually document in a care plan, such as working out the most useful ways to help patients cope positively with their anxiety or as a means of giving detailed planning for an aspect of health education or patient teaching.

Case study – Mrs Lampeter

For example, when trying to devise an aromatherapy plan for Mrs Lampeter we were able to use the Special Intervention sheet to work through the main issues. The Special Intervention was based around using touch in the form of massage with essential oils to help her feel more positive about recovery. We had talked about the oils and massage previously to this. The primary nurse was keen on the idea and asked if something could be worked out with Mrs Lampeter.

This demonstrates the confidence of the primary nurse: although she did not have the knowledge and skills, she enabled an associate nurse to utilize her skills and demonstrated that she was happy to be taught basic massage techniques by the associate nurse. Mrs Lampeter was asked what she would describe as her main problems and she listed sickness, aching in the legs, pain in the abdomen and not being able to sleep.

The Special Intervention sheet was used as a means of nurse and patient education, to list these concerns and then to work out a blend of oils that would help relieve the problems. The sheet showed the workings out in arriving at the blend and concentration of oils to be used in a leg massage. It also showed how the oils were tested on Mrs Lampeter for sensitivity, and how and when the massage should be carried out.

Case study – Larry

In another situation, a patient, Larry, who had Parkinson's disease and came in for respite care started to experience hallucinations. The day before, he had increased his medication and I assessed that his disturbed behaviour was probably due to toxicity from the increased medication. The GP prescribed a tranquillizer should the nurses feel it needed to be given.

I needed to reflect on how I felt about working with Larry when he was hallucinating and how Larry was feeling. I had to do this first before working out how I could best help Larry. I needed to be sure that I had no fear of working with Larry and that I could identify therapeutic interventions for helping him. I assessed that he was not a danger to himself or others and that he was safe to be in the hospital environment.

I decided that although I could give a low priority to Larry, in effect 'to leave him to get on with it' and only intervene when there was a problem, this was not the best way of helping him. Neither did I want to use the tranquillizers as this would only have been to make his behaviour easier for me to manage. I decided to spend some time with Larry to see if I could help him. I was also aware that my presence might actually cause him to become more disturbed.

I found that Larry was not further disturbed by my presence and that he seemed to seek out companionship. He used me to talk about what he felt was happening to him. From this I realized that he had some insight into the hallucinations and could be facilitated to see that they were not entirely real.

For example, he became fairly convinced that one of the other patient's visitors was stealing something and that was why they were leaving the building. Larry wanted to follow them until the police arrived. I was able to facilitate him to understand that this was not happening as he had initially perceived it to be. I did this by using questions that required him to work out the logic of what was happening. At no time did I feel it was right to simply tell him he was imagining things. I had assumed that Larry was not so disturbed as to have lost his problem-solving skills. This then led Larry to identify that he was having 'dreams', thus demonstrating that he had some insight into his situation.

I felt it was appropriate to write this up as a Special Intervention. The interaction strategies were very important and needed to be communicated to other nurses so that they could build on my work, rather than work out all the dynamics for themselves each time they came on duty. This type of intervention could not be prescribed as it involved some reflection-in-action, or working out what to do as you went along. The Special Intervention became:

> Larry is experiencing some 'dreams' which are causing him to feel distressed. During his dreams Larry is fully awake. How can we best work with Larry to help him through these dreams? Please make a note of any interventions or strategies that seem to help Larry.

I then documented the interventions and strategies I had found useful. I would expect the primary nurse to review the intervention and amend it as appropriate. All nurses who work with Larry would add helpful interventions and strategies as well as commenting on the usefulness of previously written ones, thus testing them further in practice and evaluating their effectiveness.

The stress of using the Burford model

Thinking about this topic I identified four main areas of stress from the perspective of a full-time associate nurse. I feel that it is important to highlight these to create a balance in the chapter since the previous ideas have been so positive!

Involvement

The first area I identified as stressful was the involvement demanded from the practitioner in nurse–patient/family relationships. To be therapeutic involves two-way sharing and the emotional energy this can demand from the practitioner can be very draining. If each nurse has only a finite amount of energy which has to be shared between work-life and home-life, and great demands are placed upon them at work, then home-life can suffer and vice versa. For example:

> Fred was admitted to Burford hospital following cerebral infarcts which left him functionally blind and confused. His wife, Agnes, was distraught by these events – they had always been totally dependent upon each other, having had no children – and she was exhibiting signs that she could not see a future without Fred. For this reason she only left the hospital to sleep and expected intensive input from nursing staff all day and night which due to other patient demands was impossible.
>
> Agnes's stress levels meant that she had unrealistic expectations of the input we could give, both physically and emotionally. She would interrupt lunch breaks, telephone calls, work with other patients, and even impinge on off-duty time, for example, stopping my car as I left the car park to go home and telephoning staff at home.

Reflecting on how this affected myself and listening to other staff talking it was obvious that Agnes demanded so much of our energy at work that home-life was suffering: partners were becoming irritable because they did not want to hear, again, about Agnes and Fred; social life was suffering as few of us had the inclination to do much except sleep once we had left work. Consequently our working practice began to suffer as resentment for Agnes grew.

The model demands that we work holistically and therapeutically with patients and so when my energy reserves run low feelings of guilt emerge as I am aware that I am not working as I should.

Primary nursing

Although this area of stress is often easily resolved due to team dynamics, I feel it is appropriate to highlight it briefly. The stress relates to both primary nursing and the BNDU model: if I admit a patient in the absence of the primary nurse and begin to build a therapeutic relationship, do I relinquish this on the return of the primary nurse? If I do I may feel cheated and undervalued and if I do not the primary nurse is placed in a dilemma of role definition.

As I stated, however, this is usually overcome due to good working relationships within the nursing team: if I feel strongly about the relationship I have established, the primary nurse will often enable me to be primary nurse to that individual with much support.

Access to one's own feelings

The reflective nature of the model encourages accessing one's own feelings, and although this is usually a positive stressor, at times it can be negative since awareness of feelings leads to action upon them which may create further stress as the actions may not be easy to carry out. For example:

> When the behaviour of a respite patient changed such that it was causing stress for the daughter, (the main carer), I realized that I felt resentment towards the patient for upsetting the daughter. However, I did not wish to act on this and so chose the easy option of observing the patient in order to 'pick up clues'. Through reflection and supervision I realized that this was not the most therapeutic way to act and was challenged to confront the patient which was not an easy action for me as I did not wish to upset her.

Time

The model provides so much scope for good practice, but it does not provide any more hours in the day! Consequently work is 'taken home' and may interfere with relaxation. Although as an associate nurse I may not bring home practical work as the primary nurses do I still have emotional and problem-solving work I do at home.

Coping with stress

Burford's philosophy of practice articulates the essential nature and significance of the therapeutic team to reciprocate and sustain practitioners in therapeutic work. A key issue for us is to both utilize and contribute to this resource. Clearly, where work creates stress, then systems are needed to deal with it. It is not satisfactory to take it home. Yet experiences have shown that this is not always achieved as personal concerns do sometimes get in the way, and we become resentful, angry and defensive with our colleagues.

Without doubt, a key aspect of effective work is being able to give and receive support from each other. The point cannot be emphasized enough in using the BNDU model to its full potential. Yet it is not always easy to achieve this despite its 'espoused' value. We are all too human sometimes!

Creativity

As we have demonstrated, working with the model can enable nurses and their nursing to become more creative. We feel this has immense benefits for both the patient and the nurse. For patients, their care becomes more personal and more individualized. Nurses become more focused on developing therapeutic relationships with patients rather than doing things to patients (Alfano 1971). This means that the working day for nurses is organized around the needs of patients rather than around the span of duty being worked by the nurses.

We believe that in the long term more positive health outcomes can be achieved by nurses communicating effectively with patients than by getting through the jobs that need to be done. This is not to say that 'basic' aspects of care are neglected. It is important that patients' needs for physical care are also met.

In the BNDU model we are continuously striving to become creative in our work with patients and families. This is not always easy as we are constrained by socialization processes in nursing (Melia 1987). Traditional nursing education socializes nurses into acceptance – acceptance of rules and regulations, of policies and procedures. It is often problematic for nurses to break free of these constraints and move towards therapeutic patient-centred care which requires nurses to think critically for themselves.

This is especially so for lone nurses trying to change their own practice within a team of nurses who continue to practise in traditional nurse-centred ways. Creativity must be acknowledged and accepted by a team of nurses for it to become effective in patient care. The relationships between the nurses must also be conducive to creativity. Nurses need to trust each other and not worry because they are not all doing the same things in the same way.

Becoming creative is clearly a learning process which incorporates an understanding of different types of knowledge. Becoming sensitive to problems, recognizing disharmonies and making guesses suggests that knowledge other than research-based scientific knowledge is of value. This further validates the usefulness of constructed knowledge as described by Belenky *et al.* (1986) and sources of knowledge described as aesthetic and personal by Carper (1978).

As Vaughan (1992) states, aesthetic knowledge can be referred to as the art of nursing. It incorporates elements of intuition and involves the carrying out of an assimilation of multiple sources of knowledge with relevance to a particular context at a particular time. Personal knowing is about developing self-awareness and self-understanding. We have found that reflection can facilitate the development of self-knowing. This is one of the reasons we emphasize the use of reflection and reflective techniques in the BNDU model and generally in our practice as it further supports our work with patients.

Conclusions

We have attempted to give an insight into the use of the BNDU by us as associate nurses. We have shown how the model can be used as a framework and a guide in practice, and rather than constraining our practice it enables us to practice in more patient-centred ways using more creative nursing strategies and interventions. Learning to work with the model and learning to work with patients requires time, energy and commitment from us as individuals and from our team.

References

Alfano, G. (1971) Healing or caretaking – which will it be? *Nursing Clinics of North America*, **6**(2), 273–80.

Belenky, M.F., Clinchy, B.M., Goldberger, N.R. & Tarule, J.M. (1986) *Women's Ways of Knowing*. Basic Books, New York.

Berne, E. (1964) *Games People Play: The Psychology of Human Relationships*. Penguin, London.

Callahan, S. (1988) The role of emotion in ethical decision-making. Hastings Center Report, **18** 9–14.

Carper, B.A. (1978) Fundamental Patterns of Knowing in Nursing. *Advances in Nursing Science*, **1**(1), 13–23.

Johns, C.C. (1991) The Burford Nursing Development Unit holistic model of nursing practice. *Journal of Advanced Nursing*, **16**, 1090–98.

Johnstone, D.E. (1989) Some thoughts on nursing. *Clinical Nurse Specialist*, **3**, 1–4.

Manthey, M. (1973), Primary nursing is alive and well in the hospital. *American Journal of Nursing*, **73**(1), 83–7.

Manthey, M. (1980) *The Practice of Primary Nursing*. Blackwell Scientific Publications, Oxford.

Melia, K. (1987) *Learning and Working – The Occupational Socialisation of Nursing*. Tavistock Publications, London.

Pearson, A. (1988) *Primary Nursing: Nursing in the Oxford and Burford Nursing Development Units*. Chapman & Hall, London.

Salvage, J. (1990), Introduction. In: *Models for Nursing*, 2 (eds J. Salvage & B. Kershaw), Scutari Press, Harrow, Middlesex.

Vaughan, B. (1992), The nature of nursing knowledge. In: *Knowledge for Nursing Practice*, (eds K. Robinson & B. Vaughan). Butterworth-Heinemann, Oxford.

Webb, C. (1992) The use of the first person in academic writing: objectivity, language and gatekeeping. *Journal of Advanced Nursing*, **17**, 747–52.

Editor's commentary

Kate Butcher's case study of Bert illustrates how staff come to label patients as 'difficult' as a means of dealing with their anxieties. Kate illustrates her responsibility as an associate nurse to confront these restricted attitudes from her colleagues and so emphasizes the associate role as being creative in its own right rather than merely a passive follower of prescribed care. In fact this chapter constantly reinforces the significance of this 'creative' stance for the development of personal growth and effective caring and how the BNDU model facilitates this.

Kate explores her personal development through three case studies. She suggests that a lack of structure within the BNDU assessment may cause difficulties for students and newly qualified staff. Kate's stress is a reflection of her inexperience and the somewhat invidious position she found herself in at Burford at that time. Ideally this situation should not have been allowed to develop.

This observation is also a reflection of how nurses are educated within colleges of nursing and socialized on the wards into a stereotyped response to viewing and assessment of the patient. As a result, when faced with alternate ways of looking at the world they are at a loss as to how to proceed and become stressed.

The case studies in this chapter highlight the value of supervision and how this enabled Kate to identify, confront and resolve the contradictions between her beliefs and the way she practised. Of particular value were the cue questions that focus on the patient's and practitioner's own feelings and how these feelings interface within the care situation. Through her case studies, Kate reinforces the significant part emotions play in decision-making (Callahan 1988) and becoming involved with patients, both key interventions in using the BNDU model.

Jan Dewing's experiences show how her sensitivity to her own feelings and to the patient resulted in her ability to identify and respond to need rather than imposing hasty interpretations. The message that the patient must have received from Jan was the perception of a sensitive nurse who demonstrated genuine concern for the patient as a person at this strange and frightening time. Jan sets up the potential for the trusting relationship necessary for therapeutic caring.

The associate nurse plays a key role in responding to the patient. They spend as much time with the patient as does the primary nurse and as such this role must be valued. It is interesting to compare the accounts of Lyn Sutherland and Roger Cowell (Chapters 3 and 4 respectively) with this account. Lyn's focus is on herself and her relationships with her patients whereas Roger is more expansive and open to influences. This reflects the development of collegial relationships between primary nurses and associate nurses necessary for associate nurses to feel they have a valued and acknowledged role in being creative and responsive with patients, and the need to confront primary nurses with any sense of 'owning' the patient and dominating the care the patient receives.

Thus the primary nurse must be able to give and receive feedback in mutually supportive ways, and allow, as expressed within the Burford philosophy for practice, the development of the therapeutic team as a whole.

Chapter 6
The BNDU Model in Use at the Oxford Community Hospital: The Case of Eva

Brendan McCormack, Carol McCaffrey and Susan Booker

This chapter has three main intentions:

- To utilize the supporting themes of the BNDU holistic model of nursing in order to describe the context in which the model was used in a specific practice environment.
- To highlight a particular case to describe the utility of the model in practice.
- Using a particular theoretical framework, to offer a critical analysis of the appropriateness of the model for practice.

This case study describes the care given to a particular patient using the BNDU model of nursing and offers a critique of the usefulness of the model for practice. The model is not one that is widely used in the particular practice area, but is one that practitioners are becoming more familiar with.

The setting in context

The four key components of the philosophy for practice as described by Johns (1991) and from which the BNDU holistic model was developed are:

- External environment of care
- Internal environment of care
- Social viability
- The nature of care

Environment of care

The emphasis of the BNDU holistic model is practice and because practice is rooted in an environment which is unstable and unpredictable then the need to 'capture the reality of practice and the beliefs and values of the practitioners' is paramount. This tension between the espoused ideology and the ideology in practice and its resultant effects on patient care has been recently documented by Ahmed and Kitson (1992). The authors concluded that the tension between the two ideologies led to inconsistent and discontinuous care patterns. It is not new for nurse theorists to address environment issues in their development of nursing models, (for example, Roper *et al.* 1990; Roy 1989; Orem 1985). Indeed Roper *et al.* (1990, p.30) state:

'Environmental factors cannot be considered in isolation; they are related to physical, psychological and sociocultural ... and also to politicoeconomic factors...'

However, in addressing environmental issues Roper *et al.* (1990) discuss such topics as the atmosphere, sunrays, light rays, sound waves and atmospheric components. While these are certainly important factors in our everyday living and our health status, they are not the issues that immediately come to the mind of the practitioner in everyday practice (Melia 1990; Benner & Wrubel 1989). The BNDU model attempts to address more local environment issues. These will now be discussed in the context of the authors' areas of practice.

External environment of care

The external environment relates to the context and function of the particular nursing practice (Johns 1991), and the philosophy must be relevant to the context of where the care is carried out (Johns 1990).

Oxford Community Hospital (OXCOMM) is one of eleven community hospitals in the community unit of Oxfordshire Health Authority. Founded in 1984 with just ten beds it was one of the first urban community hospitals in the country. In 1988 the hospital expanded and now has the capacity to cater for up to twenty-four inpatients and eight day patients.

Unlike the other community hospitals, OXCOMM is not an independent building, but is situated within the structure of a large general hospital. The hospital serves a predominantly elderly population (although not designated an elderly care area) in a local environment with a range of services from rehabilitation, respite care for the chronically sick, care of the dying and day hospital assessment and treatment. These services are centred around an operational philosophy which states:

'... Oxford Community Hospital should function as an integral part of the community health services with an emphasis on the maintenance and resettlement of people in their "home" environment.' (Oxford Community Hospital, unpublished observations)

This approach to service delivery is consistent with that recommended in Tucker's (1987) research whereby:

'The community hospital serves the community and is served by the community'.

Indeed, the NHS Health Advisory Service (NHS 1991) recognizes that the community hospitals of Oxfordshire are ideally placed to be developed as:

'... multi-disciplinary, multi-agency resource centres with full access for local residents, sub-serving the social, physical and mental health needs of elderly people'.

The hospital is actively involved in developing an outreach philosophy and the strengthening of links between primary and secondary care.

Internal environment of care

The internal environment is concerned with issues such as relationships between nurses and with other health professionals (Johns 1991).

The organization of nursing at OXCOMM is based on the philosophy of primary nursing. Each patient admitted is allocated a named nurse, known as a primary nurse, who is responsible for the coordination of care for that patient within the multidisciplinary team. This organizational philosophy has been in practice since the inception of the unit and is an established ideology among practitioners. However, issues relating to role ambiguity and confusion are evident in the hospital, and, due to the number of staff employed and the irregular hours worked, practical difficulties in maintaining open and honest lines of communication exist (B.G. McCormack, unpublished observations). Behaviour which characterizes this culture includes:

- giving and receiving feedback, which creates an impression of authenticity but which does not in fact provide it
- maintaining interpersonal diplomacy
- withholding feelings

- suppressing anger
- hurt, suspicion and mistrust (McCormack, 1993).

Because of this culture, therapeutic interaction between staff is problematic and these behaviours are consistent with those described by Johns (1990) in his concept of the 'harmonious team'.

The concept of therapeutic reciprocity is central to the BNDU model, where the relationships between staff need to match those between the nurse and patient (Johns 1991). An essential component of therapeutic reciprocity is self-knowledge. Egan (1990) suggests that effective helpers undertake the lifelong task of fulfilling the Ancient Greek injunction, 'Know thyself'. It is not enough to know the client in the helping relationship; it is essential to understand one's own assumptions, beliefs, values, strengths and weaknesses and the ways in which these permeate interactions with patients. The cue question, 'How does this person make me feel?', implores the nurses to address their values and assumptions and recognize the importance of these when engaging in an authentic relationship with patients.

As yet no unit philosophy exists to act as the cornerstone for the practice of nursing according to an explicitly stated set of beliefs and values. Inglesby (1992) is critical of nursing using the word 'philosophy' in this way. She suggests that the only laudable way to use the word is in the description of philosophical issues that might have influenced nurses'/nursing's beliefs and in the area of moral philosophy.

While purists may appreciate the relevance of this criticism, it could be argued that the present approach allows nurses to use the medium of their beliefs and values to develop a philosophy for nursing which identifies humanistic–scientific factors (Watson 1985) as central to the practice of nursing. Watson suggests that the recognition of the humanity of the individual is central to the nurse–patient relationship, whereby individuals 'make public' their value systems and feelings in order to achieve reciprocity and authenticity in the relationship.

As this practice setting is in a transitional period, the beliefs and values of practitioners are emerging and philosophical issues relating to the uniqueness of the individual, therapeutic use of self, the nature of care, intuitive creativity and individual potential are all concepts that are being explored through practice. These beliefs and values can be seen to be compatible with those expressed in the BNDU model.

A programme of support is established in the form of organizational developments centred around contract learning, clinical supervision and performance review, in order to facilitate the integration of humanistic principles in caring and the complex learning that this involves.

Social viability

Social viability relates to the value of nursing to the society it serves. Implicit in this approach is the value of nursing models.

Practitioners at OXCOMM utilize Roper, Logan and Tierney's (1990) model of nursing to guide their practice. While this model has been adapted to suit the particular practice setting, it is often criticized by practitioners for not fulfilling the role they require. Such comments as, 'We don't like the "boxes" approach to assessment', 'There is more to life than activities of living', and 'I feel committed to complete all the sections even though they may not be relevant', demonstrate this dissatisfaction.

Meleis (1991) warns against unnecessary assessment or intervention that could be more effectively achieved by other members of the health care team. This unnecessary assessment leads to the intrusive and mechanistic nature of the assessment process which is commonly expressed by practitioners in this setting. The model is seen by practitioners as not fitting easily with the more humanistic beliefs and values which they espouse.

The model of nursing is based on what Roper *et al.* (1990) describe as a model of living, which encapsulates five elements:

- activities of living
- life-span
- dependence/independence continuum
- factors influencing activities of living
- individuality in living.

The authors postulate that 'a model of living must offer a way of describing what "living" means'. While recognizing that most people would describe everyday activities such as eating, drinking and sleeping as essential to life, many philosophical issues of living may also be seen as important. Indeed Watson (1985) argues that:

'A humanistic–altruistic value system is a qualitative philosophy that guides one's mature life'

and it is this value system that:

'... helps one to tolerate differences and to view others through their own perceptual systems rather than through one's own'.

It is difficult to capture this individual phenomenological approach to experience within a model that focuses on body systems. The model of living does not easily transfer assessment of needs to an individualized holistic plan of care.

Roper *et al.*'s model conforms to a linear model of analysis. However, more contemporary work suggests that decision-making in nursing does not necessarily adhere to the linear model, but instead incorporates a more intuitive, holistic mode of thinking (Pyles & Stern 1983; Benner 1984; Young 1987). Furthermore, adherence to formal linear models of practice devalues intuitive knowledge as a legitimate component of scientific method and fails to recognize holistic modes of thinking (McCormack 1992). The work of Benner (1984) has initiated the re-addressing of the emphasis on linear models of thinking and problem-solving, thereby causing a shift towards more holistic modes.

The nature of care

The nature of care is primarily concerned with the relationship between the nurse and the patient within the influences and constraints of the environment (Johns 1991).

Nurses at OXCOMM place value on the individuality of the person receiving care while recognizing the problematic nature of working *with* patients. Issues relating to the complexities of preserving and under-standing patient autonomy, and patients' rights to choice, raise practical and emotional concerns for nurses. The emotional labour of care has been succinctly captured by Smith (1992) in her research with student nurses. The author concluded that emotional components of caring require formal and systematic training to manage feelings.

Egan (1990) argues that helpers who do not understand themselves can inflict a great deal of harm on their clients. Therefore, the impor-tance of nurses being 'self-aware' is paramount in an organization that centres its practice on the therapeutic nurse–patient relationship.

Nurses need to be aware of their motives for caring. Clearly there are professional motives involved, as a basic tenet of being professional is the ability to be self-regulating, i.e. reflecting on practice and re-evaluating outcomes. Through this process professional practitioners identify deficiencies in practice and organize approaches for change. The BNDU model offers the client an opportunity to be involved in this self-regulating process, as its structure and focus promotes active involvement of the patient in their care management.

It can be concluded therefore that the BNDU holistic model is appropriate for this particular practice setting. While this setting is currently developing an explicitly stated set of values and beliefs in the form of a philosophy for practice, the principles which nursing staff articulate in their practice are compatible with those expressed in this model. The articulation and cohesion of these values and beliefs is recognized as a continuous process in the development of patient-centred practice in this unit.

The model in use: case study – Eva

In this case study the implementation of the BNDU model in practice was a joint decision between the patient and her carers. The authors were functioning as joint care-givers to the patient (Eva). The relationship between the authors was of student (Carol), mentor (Sue) and teacher (Brendan). Pyles and Stern (1983) recognize that the mentor, (an experienced nurse), has a key function to play in the socialization of student nurses. The mentor acts as a teacher, adviser, counsellor and role-model for the novice nurse.

The role of the teacher is that of helping the students to identify, explore and expand on their own latent knowledge (Miller & Rew 1989) in the practice setting. The teacher facilitates the students to develop and reflect on their intuitive and objective knowledge. It is essential that the teacher is seen to 'struggle' to solve problems with the student instead of only providing answers. While recognizing the use of problem-solving through linear analysis, the learner needs to be able to look deeper at problems and recognize that not all cases and problems can fit into mechanisitic frameworks (McCormack, unpublished observations). Therefore, problem-solving strategies which focus on the question rather than the answers were employed in this case.

This approach gives further credibility to the value of feelings and beliefs in the nurse–patient relationship, thus counteracting Visintainer's (1986) view that nurses place little credibility on their feelings and beliefs – the 'soft stuff' of nursing. The work of Schon (1991) has begun the re-addressing of the essence of nursing, through the reflective process. Indeed, the assessment strategy utilized in the BNDU model can be seen to be a model of reflection in itself with its starting point the question, 'What information do I need to be able to nurse this person?'

In order to capture the essence of the relationship, sections from Carol's reflective diary are included where appropriate. This approach further legitimatizes the use of the cue questions, 'How does this person make me feel?' and 'How can I help this person?', by demonstrating the nature of the interactions that occurred in this nurse–patient relationship and their articulation through reflection.

Assessment of Eva's need for care

When Eva was admitted the decision not to read her medical notes was a conscious one, since it was preferred to let her present herself to her nurse, hence guarding against any expectations or preconceived ideas about her personality or her condition.

Assessment of Eva's needs was performed initially using Roper *et al.*'s model of nursing. While much valuable information was obtained, the process of acquiring this felt uncomfortable and intrusive for both Eva and Carol.

Reflection

The model is in my opinion very functional having used it to assess my patient. She is fortunately a very open, talkative person who enjoys talking about her problems and how she sees the future for herself and her family. In order to get around the questions in Roper's model, I needed to use open questions and encouraged her husband to participate in the assessment. The most difficult part was the assessment of sexuality. This was challenging for me, if not a little embarrassing. But my patient reassured me – 'Don't worry, I don't mind' – making me feel a little more at ease. Discussing death also proved unnerving. There was something not right about this experience.

A re-assessment of Eva's needs was performed using the BNDU holistic model of nursing.

Reflection

Instead of attempting to make underlying assumptions, the BNDU holistic model has allowed me to see Eva more in the context of her social and cultural world.

The Burford model assessment consists of one core question and a series of cue questions which tune the nurse into the philosophic concepts of the model (as opposed to the functional concepts). These questions have not been altered in any way from their original format as described by Johns (1991). While Johns asserts that the cue questions do not require specific information, the assessment process in this study is presented in this way in order to demonstrate the utility of the model.

'Who is this person?'

Eva was the youngest and sole survivor of a family of four children and she had three children of her own; two daughters and one son, who all lived nearby and visited regularly. She had been married to John for thirty-eight years and prior to her hospitalization lived with him in purpose-built accommodation in Oxfordshire. A sixty-nine year old lady, she led an independent life until her disabilities overcame her physical ability to mobilize herself independently.

'What health event has brought this person into hospital?'

The aim of Eva's stay at OXCOMM was to help her to convalesce after surgery of an abscess in her left lumbar region and to come to terms with the increasing severity of her debilitating rheumatoid arthritis. Her cavity wound was a result of her taking steroid-based medication for this thirty-year-long illness. Eva was wheelchair-bound and is a diabetic. She was fighting to regain control of her continence, with increasing success following the removal of an indwelling catheter after almost four years *in situ.*

'How must this person be feeling?'

Eva once expressed to Carol that she felt that, 'Life is just one misery'. She was depressed at times, frightened that her wound would not heal quickly and exhausted by the fatigue that her arthritis caused her and the 'energy drained' feeling that she complained of, probably due to the medication she was taking. She not only feared for her own future, but also for John's (her husband), who was very concerned about her and lonely at home without her there.

'How has this event affected this person's usual life patterns and roles?'

Eva's admission to the Oxford Community Hospital affected her usual life pattern and roles minimally, since Eva's active roles had been very limited due to her crippling arthritis. She missed and yearned for the comfort and familiarity of the surroundings of her own home, John, taking her walks and tending to her plants. Eva's residual roles in her family were very strong. She was a very communicative person who said that she was always 'ready for a chat'. She enjoyed airing her feelings, reminiscing about the past and reflecting often on the present and the uncertainty which the future held.

'How does this person make me feel?'

On the whole, Eva made us feel good; the role as her nurse was a highly rewarding and satisfying one. Eva, despite being very physically dependent, was independent in spirit and willing to participate as much as she could, in all aspects of her care. Her cooperation rarely faltered except on those days when her pain and fatigue overcame her. On such occasions Eva became passive and often self-pitying, at which time we felt great empathy towards her and a determination to cheer her up and to make her stay as comfortable as possible.

'How can I help this person?'

Eva was helped by planning the most effective health care for her. Based on an assessment of her capabilities and dependencies, the care Eva needed was both clinical (in respect of her wound) and psychological, which involved interacting with her for long periods of time and giving her continuous encouragement and reassurance.

'What is important to make this person's stay in hospital comfortable?'

- *Firstly*, management of her pain. Eva described it is a 'round the clock' problem. Her pain was multi-focal and ranged on a Raiman scale from moderate to severe. Eva often complained of pains in her back, neck and had frequent headaches.
- *Secondly*, care of her wound. Eva's wound caused her much distress, resulting in her always asking, 'How is it getting on?', when it was being redressed. She saw her wound as the main obstacle preventing her returning home; hence, it was essential that we established an honest and trusting relationship, to allow her to come to terms with the severity of her illness, using a sensitive, positive approach.
- *Thirdly*, management of her continence and bowels. Although these may not to a diagnosing clinician stand out as either of Eva's main problems, they were her main concerns, causing her much anxiety. She was prone to constipation since she did not move around very much, and as a result she felt 'so bloated'. Having recently had a four-year catheter removed, Eva was concerned about maintaining her self-esteem, and was successfully regaining control of her continence.

'What support does this person have?'

Eva's primary support person was her husband. John very proudly said, 'I do everything for her,' when at home. He did the washing, shopping and cooking, helping her up in the mornings and to bed at night.

Although John felt very capable and said he was 'very fit', he suffered from angina and was often very breathless upon coming to visit Eva. Nevertheless, he was very keen to get her back home, insisting that he could look after her with the assistance of a home-help during the week and a girl from 'Crossroads', a home care organization, at weekends. But after much talking about the practicalities of dealing with Eva's wound care and pain, John mentioned his desire to get her home less often as did Eva herself.

'How do they view the future for themselves and others?'

Eva described her present illness as 'the last straw' and often expressed that 'I just don't know what is going to happen next'. Since her operation to have her wound sutured, and with much counselling Eva had come to realize that she and John could not cope alone at home. She certainly wished to return home and to regain some of her independence, which would require a lot of willpower and motivation not only on her part but on that of her husband. She said that she did not know what she would do without John, and we got the impression that if he were gone she would give up the will to live.

Planning and giving care

Due to the patient-centred approach of the assessment process, it was deemed appropriate to use metaphors to describe the planning and implementation of care.

Following assessment of Eva's needs, a 'priorities of care' list was drawn up with Eva (Fig. 6.1), using Neuman's levels of nursing interventions as discussed in the BNDU model (Johns 1991).

Problem: 'I've had my fill of hospitals'
Focus of problem: loss of self-esteem and depression

Eva openly expressed her negative feelings about being at the Community Hospital. She said that she was sick of being in hospital and would prefer to be cared for at home where she could 'do her own thing' and be with John. In our recognition that this was impossible at present, we did realize that it was especially important for Eva's wound to heal quickly, and by giving her lots of support throughout her stay we aimed to allow her to return home as soon as possible.

Eva's admission undoubtedly had psychological and social implications for her; her removal from the home environment and her missing her husband were contributing factors.

Primary interventions
(1) Preparation of Eva for return to her own home with John as her main carer.
(2) Preparation of John for Eva's discharge home and equipping him with the necessary skills to care for her.
(3) Promotion of Eva's self-esteem by reinforcing a positive self-image while caring for her.

Secondary interventions
(1) Wound care.
(2) Control of Eva's diabetes and promotion of wound healing through the provision of adequate nutrition.
(3) Control of Eva's pain including massage.

Tertiary interventions
(1) Control of Eva's continence.
(2) Support for John in his caring role.

Fig. 6.1 Priorities of care.

Reflection

I understand the concept of the patient's experience as a crucial element of the philosophy of care. It is necessary to focus on and understand what the illness event means to Eva and her family; hence the importance of taking her assessment and viewing her as a member of the community, with a social and cultural world, and centring nursing action around her needs from a holistic perspective that recognizes the uniqueness of her personal experience.

One evening upon entering her room, we heard her say to her husband, 'I just look so awful.' He reassured her that this was not the case, but she remained unconvinced. It could be suggested therefore that she was grieving for the loss of her body image, a consequence of her deteriorating arthritis and her ever-increasing problems with mobility, resulting in her low self-esteem and lack of social roles. Either way, we recognized that time, patience and understanding were of the essence when delivering care to Eva. Having implemented this in the care plan, we felt that perhaps the carers could accept her depression as a 'natural process' of expressing her grief.

Problem: 'My back is killing me'
Focus of problem: wound care and maintenance of Eva's autonomy

The dimensions of the wound and its location contributed to the discomfort caused to Eva, especially upon physical exertion, and indeed she reiterated this on numerous occasions. 'My back is killing me,' she would often say, accounting not only for her physical discomfort but also for her depression, for which she took daily medication.

The need for Eva's wound to heal quickly required selection of a suitable dressing, since inappropriate selection can often increase pain (Thomas 1989). A thorough assessment of the wound was completed. A calcium-alginate-based ribbon dressing to pack her wound daily was used, with the knowledge that the predicted rapid and pain-free healing process employed would help Eva make a speedy recovery which would assist in improving her psychological status and increase her social roles.

Care of Eva's wound involved irrigation, assessment and redressing daily. We allowed Eva to decide the time when this procedure was performed. In doing this we felt that we were not disturbing her usual routine which was important as she felt anxious and depressed at times, and appreciation of her wanting to have a lie-in could warrant her feeling more at home and at ease during her stay. This approach was appropriate for her and Eva was able to plan her day in advance with John.

Reflection

I was reminded of this quote from Forster (1989) which reflected the complexity of preserving patient autonomy.

> When my time comes I'm not going to allow it.
> When my time comes I won't trust to mystery.
> When my time comes I will say I have had enough and go.
> That is, if my time comes like Grandma's time.
> If it is the same sort of time.
> But if it is, I won't be able to, will I?

Problem: 'Do I have to eat this?'
Focus of problem: control of Eva's diabetes and promotion of wound healing through the provision of appropriate diet

Concurrent with Eva's wound management was the need for her to be well-nourished. She was a diet-controlled diabetic and had been 'for a couple of years now'. In the knowledge that diabetes is the most common condition that may account for delayed healing of wounds due to defective carbohydrate and fat metabolism (Ross & Benditt, 1962), Eva's 'BM stix' were recorded twice daily. Ross and Benditt's study also emphasized the need for normal protein metabolism.

Following a long chat with Eva, we all agreed that she should commence a high protein diet. Eva had complained on several occasions about her food: 'It's awful,' she said. This helped her accept a special diet, and she was pleased to have special soups and yoghurts sent from the kitchen, in addition to the sugar-free extras (drinks, fruit and sweets) brought by John nearly every evening. When asked how she was eating she replied, 'Very well. The food seems to have improved'.

We did feel the need to reinforce Eva's nutrition patterns however. Following discussion with her, we emphasized the importance of her continuing with this regime on her return home, knowing that the slightest possibility of readmission would upset Eva and John a great deal. Both were adamant that they would stick to the present regime, John reassuring us that he would 'keep an eye on her'.

Reflection

This approach to Eva's care reinforces the importance of partnership in the nurse–patient relationship. Through focusing on the cue question, 'Who is this person?', it remained paramount to always allow Eva to take the lead in organizing her care delivery.

Problem: 'I feel so bruised and tender that life is just one misery' Focus of problem: control of Eva's pain

Parallel to and precipitated by Eva's wound care was her multi-focal pain. Indeed, Eva found any form of movement difficult and painful, especially her neck which felt so bruised and tender. It was obvious that she was in pain upon mobilizing, not only via her verbal cues but also her agonized facial expression and the gasps which seemed to take the breath from her. From Eva's perspective, it was felt that by allowing her to monitor her pain and giving her some autonomy, she would think more objectively about it, thus allowing an opportunity for all of us to set the most appropriate goals for the future. Most importantly, the mere fact that Eva could see we were taking her pain seriously could perhaps make her feel better.

Reflection

On a few occasions I have found myself in the situation where an elderly patient has complained of pain, and I have thought, 'She's looking for attention', or 'It can't be that bad!' Later I felt ashamed of myself for denying the patient their autonomy and individuality, whilst denying myself the opportunity to fulfil my role as a partner in what should be a 'mutual trust' relationship with my patient.

Eva's previous experience of pain and the anxiety that she was experiencing regarding admission to hospital were clearly associated with her pain ratings. On those days that Eva expressed feeling down or depressed, she complained of more pain. Indeed, Bond (1984) states that such anxiety can often intensify pain and this was evident with Eva.

One particular day when Eva expressed that 'Life is just one misery', her pain ratings were higher than usual and she described her pain as 'unbearable'. Hence we felt a need to spend time talking with Eva, giving her information regarding her pain and its control. The mutual trust relationship which we had established enabled more effective recognition of anxiety-evoking stimuli that were affecting her. We felt we were making contact with Eva's feelings and concerns, thereby learning from the patient and developing our clinical knowledge.

This example clearly illustrates what Benner (1984) has called situated meaning, whereby the patient does not respond to the situation solely in terms of what they have lost, but instead continues to be engaged by concerns, meanings and even a limited future (Benner & Wrubel, 1989).

Eva spoke of 'missing John', of 'feeling so useless', and had a general concern about the present and future likelihood of her recovery to full health. 'I just don't know what's going to happen to me,' she once said. By allowing John open visiting hours, and using Eva's own bed linen as well as the homely comforts of a radio and TV in her room, we felt we could make Eva more comfortable in her present surroundings and less concerned about the future.

Eva always preferred to leave her bedroom door open so she could see 'what was going on', hence often attracting the attention of a passerby, to whom she would complain of pain followed by sleepless nights. Whether or not these were due to the noisy environment (beside the nurse's station) or her Temazepan-controlled insomnia, we are not sure. Mullooly *et al.* (1988) has suggested that patients report less pain when nursed in quiet surroundings. Eva had 'settled in well now' and we felt it would have been unfair to move her to another room. We did feel though that this could be taken into consideration upon any future admissions to the unit, although Eva said she preferred the room she was in.

We found that distracting activities often seemed to be effective in controlling Eva's pain. She would sit for long periods doing a puzzle or watching TV and never talked about pain or discomfort. The family influence cannot be overlooked, however. When John came to visit, the pain behaviour increased and we often had to help him to turn her in bed. The literature suggests that this is not uncommon (Hosking & Welchew 1985); hence, we accepted it as one of Eva's characteristics.

However, not all staff were able to see it in this way and this sometimes resulted in their demonstration of controlling behaviour towards Eva.

Reflection

I found it interesting to note my feelings of protection and advocacy when this was being discussed negatively by other staff. Confronting them about their attitude was easier said than done and I often tended to just say nothing in the hope that their conversation would soon end.

In order to reduce Eva's pain during the redressing of her wound which was 'so painful', we decided a massage session might be of benefit. She expressed willingness to have her lower legs massaged using aromatherapy oils. We talked through the procedure, encouraging her to concentrate on the massage. The outcome was rewarding and Eva spoke of how much she had enjoyed the session.

Reflection

By initiating these massage sessions, I felt as if I had developed my communication skills with her, not just verbally but now non-verbally. The outcome for me was more than rewarding – she spoke on several occasions of how much she had enjoyed the sessions. I feel an outcome for both of us was a feeling of 'being cared for'. For her, the benefits were two-fold; the release of her emotions and buried feelings as she tensed muscles and aching joints were soothed, providing obvious contentment and feelings of well-being. Secondly, the attention was detracted from the wound as was mine and Eva's aim. I received feedback from other nurses that Eva asked after me and said how kind I was and how much she enjoyed my massage sessions. Making decisions about her present and future care were made easier by this relationship.

There was little doubt that Eva's pain would be ever present on her return home and it was necessary to encourage her to keep occupied as much as possible. John was very protective over her and tended to do everything for her. She missed doing the chores and went on to say, 'Now John has to do them all'. We encouraged a more participative role in her lifestyle as this could increase Eva's morale and feeling of having the pain 'under control', enabling her to play a more active role both physically and socially.

Eva said she felt 'so useless now'. Her interests were all passive ones; she enjoyed reading, watching TV and doing puzzles. She said she used to make a cake every time her son came round to see her, but was 'not able to do so now'. We found ourselves questioning her abilities. Was she physically unable or was she simply not given the initiative to take more active roles? Discussion with Eva reassured us that we could eliminate her pain as the cause of her lack of activity.

Reflection

> This I must appreciate and understand, since the threat of any potential pain would obviously prove too much, and, further, she is uncertain as to what the future holds for her; she is unsure about when she will return home, if ever she reaches a recovery state acceptable to her, where pain and immobility are not prevalent.

Problem: 'Paving the way to self-control'
Focus of problem: control of continence

Eva's concern with her bowels and her continence was hardly surprising since she had recently had a four-year indwelling catheter removed. She also suffered from constipation as a result of her poor muscle tone and limited mobility, and possibly as one of the side-effects of her medication. Eva had become very upset on a few occasions about how she 'cannot go' herself, but was willing to have an enema every two days to relieve her discomfort. Having re-established her routine, Eva began to 'go on her own', and she felt 'this is great'.

By establishing a continence programme for Eva she was 'going less often'. Initially after removal of her catheter, Eva was using her commode almost every hour, passing large amounts of urine. Later she regained control of her micturition and often did not ask for a commode for at least two hours at a time. We had to spend a lot of time educating and reassuring Eva, especially when helping her to get up in the mornings, explaining that her lack of control was to be expected, but she always just said, 'I wish I could go on my own, like everyone else'.

Evaluation of care and achieving outcomes

From a physical perspective, Eva presented us with a plethora of needs which complicated each other. However, we reached a mutually satisfying conclusion. Our aim whilst working with her was to recognize her real potential within the hospital's rehabilitation philosophy:

> 'We believe that OXCOMM should offer a rehabilitation service, based on the assumption that clients will ultimately be discharged to another setting whilst recognizing that this process may, for some people, take a long time.' (Oxford Community Hospital, unpublished observations)

Throughout her care programme, Eva's holistic care needs were met and no need was viewed in isolation. The BNDU model offered the opportunity to achieve this through its focus on philosophical concepts rather than activities of living.

However, the model does appear to lack any structural direction for the planning of care and evaluation of outcomes, other than stating that the model:

> '... rejects any determinism that manifests itself by stating goals in terms of what the patient will achieve without patient involvement.' (Johns 1991).

The setting of goals in this model does take a patient-centred approach, so therefore one assumes that it is the patient's perspective that determines when goals have been achieved. This phenomenological approach to assessment and care planning is one that as yet would be unfamiliar to most nurses, and may be one of the reasons why this model may be rejected by practitioners without appropriate support to facilitate this cultural and attitudinal change. Without this cultural paradigm shift, practitioners may never achieve the full potential of the model, by relying on linear approaches to problem identification rooted in a functional perspective.

Evaluation of the outcomes of Eva's care centred round a daily evaluation of the objectives of care compared to Eva's long-term objectives. Eva's own comments were used as part of this evaluation process and agreement was reached when changes in the direction of care were required. This process facilitated the communication of Eva's psycho-social needs and minimized the regression towards evaluation of physical care centred on activities of daily living. If patient autonomy is to be really respected, then it would seem appropriate for nurses to legitimize the value of patients' comments, interactions and discussions by utilizing their actual words rather than our interpretations of them.

Critique of the BNDU model as experienced in this particular practice area

The debate about the usefulness or not of nursing models is one that continues to preoccupy theoreticians and the nursing press. Indeed, in the pursuit of academia, nursing models have been used as the foundation for the development of theoretical principles. While the majority of these theoretical advancements fall into the conceptual model category (Kristjanson *et al.* 1987), their usefulness in guiding practice has been limited. Many of these models require further exploration of their espoused theoretical principles and their relationship and relevance to professional practice.

Evaluation of theory is an essential component of nursing practice and of knowledge development (Meleis 1991). A comprehensive framework is offered by Meleis for the evaluation of theory in nursing. This framework will be utilized to critique the model and identify development issues.

Clarity

The BNDU holistic model of nursing practice clearly articulates its underlying concepts, values and beliefs. These have been developed from practice with a focus on the articulation of internal beliefs and values. This focus arose from the belief that the imposition of external philosophy is conceptually problematic due to its potential conflict with practitioners' own beliefs and values.

The BNDU model in itself poses a similar problem, as without the articulation of a practice area's beliefs and values the model is difficult to integrate in practice. The case study of Eva highlights that the model is suitable on an individual level when a similar ideology is espoused. However, in order for its process to be accepted on a wider scale, cultural beliefs and values of the hospital would need to be explicitly stated, in order to create a shift towards more patient-centred practice. The experience of using this model suggests that it can assist this process as it offers direction for development to the practitioner. As such the model can encapsulate the collective beliefs and values of a group of practitioners, while freeing the individual practitioner from the shackles of conformity to a set of values that they may not espouse.

Consistency

Meleis (1991) describes consistency as the degree to which congruence exists between the different components of a theory. The BNDU model would appear to be consistent in its approach and the core and cue questions offer clear direction for both the assessment and organization of care. The humanistic and holistic concepts articulated in the model are reflected throughout the assessment process. However, the lack of structure in goal-setting could be problematic for the widespread adoption of this framework.

The concept of 'therapeutic interventions' would appear to require further exploration and clarification within this model, due to the weakness of the approach to evaluation. Johns (1991) asserts that the word 'therapeutic' refers to nursing action for the benefit of the patient within a focus of patient-centred needs. Hockey (1991) argues that the way in which one views the possibilities of therapeutic nursing, or what one identifies as the activity of therapeutic nursing, clearly depends on one's interpretation of it. If this is the case, then the BNDU model offers an enormous challenge to nurses and nursing and places even greater importance on the explicit statement of values and beliefs in nursing.

Many of the principles explicated in this model are appropriate to our area of practice, due to similarities in the nature of the service and patient focus. The philosophical beliefs are compatible with those of practitioners in OXCOMM and to this end the model may act as a useful tool to guide the articulation of these beliefs and values in the form of a philosophy.

Simplicity

The underlying concepts of the BNDU holistic model are relatively simple to understand and implement in practice. Chinn and Jacobs (1987) argue for simplicity in theory, but caution against simplicity in untested theory.

The model could be seen to be deceptively simple in its construction, as many of the underlying principles are complex and problematic to implement in practice due to internal and external organizational constraints. Principles such as holism, reciprocity and the notion of 'working with' are concepts that are not yet understood by nurses and indeed are often negated due to attitudinal and organizational constraints.

However, the model is easy to describe and uses language that is familiar to nurses. For this reason the model has the potential to act as a framework to aid the development of nursing practice and the articulation of therapeutic patient outcomes.

Usefulness

Some would suggest that the whole issue of nursing models has served a negative purpose in the advancement of nursing knowledge (Melia 1990; Robinson 1990) and has detracted from the real issues in nursing, i.e. the theory–practice relationship.

Meleis (1991) takes a more objective approach to the issue of nursing models and theory development and suggests that nursing is in a state of transition from that of practice, with its focus on routine and sub-servience, through the education and administration and research stages, to the present position of theory, where the development of nursing knowledge rooted in practice is paramount. Meleis (1991) suggests that contrary to other evolutionary or revolutionary developments, nursing progress seems to have charted its own path with previous rejected ideas being accepted at later stages.

A clear example of this lies within the BNDU model, whereby the concept of environment is central to the model's focus – a concept that was widely discussed by Nightingale and which was subsequently rejected by positivist science. It is within this development of 'theory of practice' (Jarvis 1992) that this model is firmly rooted and applied in the case study of Eva.

Meleis (1991) suggests that a theory should be useful in all areas of nursing including practice, research, education and administration. The BNDU holistic model has the potential to be useful in all these areas of nursing. Through the use of this model it has been possible to identify areas which need development in this practice setting. The importance of developing a philosophy for practice is one such area, as is the need to address organizational issues which negate against patient-centred practice. This perhaps is the greatest asset of the model.

Conclusions

The implementation of this model in practice has proven to be a challenge conceptually and emotionally. We felt drawn closer to the patient through the assessment process and the patient-centred approach to implementing the care programme.

While no deliberate attempt was made to alter the structure of the model for the purpose of this exercise, further work with the model through the articulation of the philosophy for practice will no doubt raise challenges that will need to be explored. This dynamic approach is refreshing as it enables the model to 'come alive' in the practice setting and grow and develop with patients' and practitioners' experience.

Indeed, as Meleis (1991, p.147) suggests:

'As we nurture and support our emerged identity, we need to support more coherent approaches to knowledge development; ones that encompass knowing, understanding and caring; ones that support the development of models for knowledge development congruent with our mission.'

Postscript

Since the writing of this chapter, Eva has died. She spent the remaining weeks before her death with her family and friends at OXCOMM. We thank her and her family for allowing us to write about her care and for the privilege of knowing her.

References

Ahmed, L. & Kitson, A.L. (1992) *The role of the health care assistant within a professional nursing culture.* Institute of Nursing, Oxford.

Benner, P. (1984) *From Novice to Expert: Excellence and power in clinical nursing practice.* Addison–Wesley Publishing Company, Menlo Park, California.

Benne, P. & Wrubel, J. (1989) *The Primacy of Caring: Stress and coping in health and illness.* Addison–Wesley Publishing Company, Menlo Park, California.

Bond, M.R. (1984) *Pain: Its nature, analysis and treatment.* Churchill Livingstone, Edinburgh.

Chinn, P.L. & Jacobs, M.K. (1987) *Theory and Nursing: A Systematic Approach,* 2nd edn. C.V. Mosby, St. Louis.

Egan, G. (1990) *The Skilled Helper: A Systematic Approach to Effective Helping.* Brooks/Cole Publishing Company, California.

Forster, M. (1989) *Have the men had enough?* Chatto & Windus, London.

Hockey, L. (1991) Foreword. In *Nursing As Therapy,* (eds R. McMahon & A. Pearson). Chapman & Hall, London.

Hosking, J. & Welchew, E. (1985) *Post-operative Pain: Understanding its nature and how to treat it.* Faber & Faber, London.

Inglesby, E. (1992) Values and philosophy of nursing – the dynamic of change? In: *Nursing Care: The challenge to change,* (eds M.J. Jolley & G. Brykczynska). Edward Arnold, London.

Jarvis, P. (1992) Reflective practice and nursing. *Nurse Education Today,* **12,** 174–81.

Johns, C.C. (1990) Autonomy of primary nurses: the need to both facilitate and limit autonomy in practice. *Journal of Advanced Nursing,* **15,** 886–94.

Johns, C.C. (1991) The Burford Nursing Development Unit holistic model of nursing practice. *Journal of Advanced Nursing,* **16,** 1090–98.

Kristjanson, L.J., Tamblyn, R. & Kuypers, J.A. (1987) A model to guide development and application of multiple nursing theories. *Journal of Advanced Nursing,* **12,** 523–29.

McCormack, B.G. (1992) Intuition: concept analysis and application to curriculum development. Part 1. *Journal of Clinical Nursing,* **1,** 339–44.

McCormack, B.G. (1993) Intuition: concept analysis and application to curriculum development. Part 2. *Journal of Clinical Nursing,* **2,** 11–17.

Meleis, A.I. (1985) *Theoretical Nursing: Development and Progress.* J.B. Lippincott Company, Philadelphia.

Melia, K. (1990) (opposing the motion) Clinical Nursing Debates 1990 – Nursing models: enhancing or inhibiting practice? *Nursing Standard,* **5**(11), 34–40.

Miller, V. & Rew, L. (1989) Analysis and Intuition: the need for both in nurse education. *Journal of Nursing Education,* **28**(2), 84–6.

Mullooly, V.M., Levin, A.F. & Feldman, H.R. (1988) Music soothes post-operative pain and anxiety. *Journal of New York State Nurses Association,* **19**(3), 4–7.

National Health Service Health Advisory Service Department of Health & Social Services Inspectorate (1991) *Report on services for mentally ill people and elderly people in the Oxfordshire Health District.* HAS/SSI(91)MI/E.63, HMSO, London.

Orem, D.E. (1980) *Nursing Concepts of Practice.* McGraw-Hill Book Company, New York.

Pyles, S.H. & Stern, P.N. (1983) Discovery of nursing gestalt in critical care nursing: the importance of the gray gorilla syndrome. *Image: The Journal of Nursing Scholarship,* **15**(2), 51–7.

Robinson, K. (1990) Nursing models – the hidden costs. *Surgical Nurse,* **11**, 13.

Roper, N., Logan, W.W. & Tierney, A.J. (1980) *The Elements of Nursing.* Churchill Livingstone, Edinburgh.

Ross, R. & Benditt, E.D. (1962) Wound Healing and Collagen Formation. *Journal of Cell Biology,* **12**, 531–33.

Roy, C.S. (1989) The Roy Adaptation Model: The Definitive Statement. In: *Conceptual Models For Nursing Practice.,* (ed. J.P. Riehl-Sisca). Appleton & Lange, California.

Schon, D. (1991) *The Reflective Practitioner,* Basic Books, New York.

Smith, P. (1992) *The Emotional Labour of Nursing: Its impact on interpersonal relations, management and the educational environment in nursing.* MacMillan Education, Basingstoke.

Thomas, S. (1989) Pain and Wound Management. *Community Outlook,* **12**, 11–15.

Tucker, H. (1987) *The role and function of community hospitals.* King's Fund, London.

Visintainer, M.A. (1986) The nature of knowledge and theory in nursing. *Image: The Journal of Nursing Scholarship,* **18**(2), 32–8.

Watson, J. (1985) *Nursing: The Philosophy and Science of Caring.* Colorado Associated University Press, Boulder, Colorado.

Young, C.E. (1987) Intuition and nursing process. *Holistic Nursing Practice,* **1**(3), 52–62.

Editor's commentary

The use of metaphors captures the quality of the patient's concerns more vividly than nursing 'diagnosis' and enables others continuing the patient's care to immediately sense and tune themselves into the essential nature of the patient's concern. In constructing appropriate metaphors, the practitioner is interpreting the patient's concerns in ways that are meaningful for them. By checking the metaphor with the patient this understanding can be validated. Usually the metaphor is a paraphrase of the patient's own words and hence makes immediate sense.

Through reflection Carol McCaffrey illustrates how caring can become a mutual process and how this led her to discover satisfaction in her caring for the patient Eva. Carol learnt to let go of her need to control Eva. Indeed, any attempts to control Eva's needs would have been counter-productive with regard to her vulnerable emotions at this time, which in turn would have undermined the attempts to manage her more physical symptoms.

This case study clearly relates the holistic nature of the patient's concerns. Although Carol manages to tease these out as discrete 'problems', in reality they merge together within Eva's illness experience. By accepting the patient within a holistic framework, Carol recognizes that the issue of greatest concern to Eva is her need to be at home and her subsequent state of mind. This becomes the unifying theme for her care.

The issue of 'the lack of structure [in the BNDU model] in goal setting could be problematic for the widespread adoption of this framework' and the suggestion that this leads to a 'weakness of evaluation' reflect traditional thinking within the nursing process framework that has encouraged linear decision-making processes. The truth is that nurses cling to the nursing process as a form of pseudo-science delusion. In truth, experienced nurses do not make decisions or set nursing goals in such a way.

As the authors identify, the use of the model requires a reorientation to a holistic and phenomenological perspective towards practice. In this way goals are not pre-determined, they are negotiated within the context of the situation. The process of negotiation enables nurses to draw on sources of knowledge to influence goal setting. In essence there is no goal setting structure within such an approach. However, the reflective nature of the BNDU model, as illustrated in this chapter, enables attention to be paid to experience and through experience to reflexively apply this knowledge to subsequent experiences.

As such, the most significant source of knowledge in setting goals and choosing appropriate interventions is personal knowledge. This is not a random knowledge based on tradition, but a systematic, dynamic and reflexive form of knowledge that has personal meaning in which 'scientific' or empirical knowledge has become assimilated. Through the use of the BNDU model and reflective practice this personal knowledge is developed as practitioners learn to pay attention to and learn through their lived experiences.

Chapter 7
Applying the BNDU Model in an Acute Medical Unit

Robert Garbett

The descriptions of the use of the model in the previous chapters have been restricted to community hospital settings. This chapter is an account of practitioners considering the use of the BNDU model as a framework for practice in an acute medical unit. How the model stands up in an acute care setting is a challenging question.

This chapter is also an account of a journey which is far from complete. It started with the need to provide practice settings for students of nursing that would reflect and complement the theoretical input that they received (Garbett 1993). The nursing team of 7e have progressed from a medical model orientation to considering the potential of nursing as an independent therapeutic agent as well as an interdependent part of hospital health care. Primary nursing has been adopted as an organizational vehicle for nursing work and has been adapted to suit the demands of acute nursing where the average patient stay is about five days.

A conceptual model for nursing, Orem's Self Care Deficit model (Orem 1991) was adopted along the way. It was chosen on the basis that it most closely reflected the beliefs and values articulated by the ward team at that time. Latterly, practice on the ward has demonstrated an evolution in the team's thinking. Hence this consideration of the possibilities of the BNDU model for use in an acute medical setting.

Exploring the value of the BNDU model is one strand of work being undertaken by the 7e Nursing Development Unit (NDU) (supported by the King's Fund Centre) within the overall aim of increasing the consistency and utility of practices related to nursing process. To this end, exploratory work has been undertaken to discover the needs of the ward's nursing team with regard to establishing a consistent philosophical underpinning to practice which will be represented by practices consistent with that philosophy. In this chapter an examination of the arguments concerning the use of models for practice is followed by a critique of the current 7e nursing philosophy with emphasis on its congruence with concepts contained within the BNDU model. Possible adaptations of the model for use in acute medicine are suggested together with examples of application from the author's practice.

Using models in practice

Since the early 1980s various nursing models have risen to a degree of prominence in the UK. Most of these have come from the USA, the most notable exception being Roper, Logan and Tierney's (1980) Activities of Living Model. Generally speaking, nursing models have been deductively derived from extant theory from the natural and social sciences. Various nurse theorists (for example, Roy (Roy & Andrews 1991) and Orem (1991)) mention that their own practice influenced their work, but there is little evidence to suggest that the most popularly adopted models have been derived inductively from the experience of practice.

While the various models of nursing may have something to offer to nursing practice, and there exists no conclusive proof that they do (Chapman 1990), the world of practice erects a number of barriers between the idealization and practice of nursing (Miller 1985). Nursing models have been adopted without question, instead of as a tool to be used critically (Gordon 1984; Lister 1987). It has been suggested that, for practising nurses, the adoption of nursing models has proved restrictive rather than facilitative to practice (Gordon 1984; B. Price, unpublished observations). It has been argued that fundamental to the problems associated with models is the fact that they are not adequately shaped by practice (Benner & Wrubel 1989). Another frequently cited barrier to the use of models is that of the use of difficult language in describing the concepts within them (Gordon 1984; Gruending 1985; Miller 1985). Nurses in the UK using models originating in North America have discovered that such models are in some ways culturally inappropriate to practice in the NHS (Wright 1986; Draper 1990).

On 7e, Orem's Self Care Deficit model was adopted during a period of fundamental change on the ward. It was chosen because it most closely matched the views of the ward team as contained in the ward philosophy at that time (Fig. 7.1). Its adoption was initially organized thoroughly and systematically. A package was written to help new members of staff understand it.

Current members of the ward team were asked for their views about various nursing process issues, including some questions about the use of models. The majority of the team named Orem as the model used on the ward. However, the extent to which this meant the strategy or the

Every person is a unique individual with social, psychological and physical needs who should be allowed to make informed choices should they so wish. They may like their families and friends to be closely involved in their care and the nurse will respect and encourage their preferences.

Patients can expect the nurses to endeavour to provide maximum physical, psychological, social and spiritual comfort for them and their families and when appropriate to help them achieve optimum independence as soon as possible.

Nurses are part of a multidisciplinary team, working together to the benefit of patients. Success of this team depends on cooperation and good communication.

Nursing care is provided by a team of nurses of different grades, each with a unique and valuable contribution to make. The qualified nurses assess the patients to identify their nursing needs. Following an assessment, a nursing care plan is written with the patient and when appropriate their family's cooperation, for the use of all the nurses in the team. Nursing care is prescribed using up-to-date nursing knowledge and in the light of experience. Nurses are accountable for the care that they prescribe, give and evaluate. Student nurses and auxiliaries are always supported and supervised by a qualified member of the nursing team.

Knowledge enables people to look after themselves and prevent reoccurrence of illness. It is therefore the nurse's important responsibility to educate patients and their families. Provision of information during the hospital stay reduces stress.

We acknowledge the importance of continuity of care and endeavour to provide this for our patients by keeping the number of nurses looking after them to a minimum.

Nursing is a developing profession in which change is an integral part. The nurses acknowledge the need for new developments and appreciate the difficulties associated with change. Team meetings to openly discuss change and provide mutual support are held on a regular basis.

If nursing care is to be provided using a knowledge base, it is every nurses' responsibility to continue her education and share this with others. Learning opportunities are provided on the ward and staff are encouraged to attend study days when possible.

Fig. 7.1   7e ward philosophy (*circa* 1989).

concepts of 'self-care deficit' underlying the model is unclear; from such expressions as, 'I use a vague interpretation of Orem's', it seemed that it was more the former than the latter. It seemed that there was a ground swell of independent practice with individuals adapting their approach and suggesting that using a model was rigid and restrictive. Previously adopted beliefs were still influential, especially with regard to thinking around 'helping them [the patients] to be able to care for themselves'.

Partly because Orem as a model has become inadequate for use by this particular team, and partly because examination of nursing-process-related issues forms part of the development work under the auspices of the King's Fund, a period of re-evaluation is now taking place on the ward, with the Burford model as one possible contribution to developments in practice. The approach being used for current development work is influenced by action research (Greenwood 1984) and democratic, practitioner-driven change strategies (Wright 1989).

Clarke (1986) wrote:

'practical activity is primary but ... theoretical activity arises from practice and serves to modify it.'

Benner (1984) suggests that theory to guide practice is embedded with practice itself. Both theory and practice are as important as each other; theory frames the issues and guides the practitioner in where to look and what to ask. But, argue Benner and Wrubel (1989), expert practice can go beyond the current state of learning and so further enrich theory. Clinical situations are always more varied and complicated than theoretical accounts, and therefore clinical practice is an arena of inquiry and knowledge development.

Practising nurses need to learn how to recognize and develop the knowledge that they use in their practice. The work of Schon (1987) amongst others has been important here. Schon, writing about architectural practice, stresses the importance of moving away from concentration on the 'high, hard ground' of manageable problems to an understanding of the 'swampy lowlands' of the complex and imperfect world of practice. Practitioners need to develop skills of reflecting critically on the impact of their practice and changing it as necessary. Practice may then perhaps be used to challenge and refine theory by validating it within a practice setting (Chinn & Jacobs 1983). Such notions underpin the curriculum for undergraduate nurses at Oxford Brookes University (Champion 1992).

The ward philosophy

Several years after the initial development work on 7e there is once again a need to revisit the conceptual bases underpinning practice. Since decisions were made about philosophical beliefs and suitable theoretical strategies there has been a substantial turnover of staff. Those staff on the ward at present have themselves encountered different ideas and influences through undertaking courses in further education at varying levels.

The nursing model presented by Johns (1991) is founded on the unit philosophy at Burford. A preliminary step to establishing the model's suitability for adoption on 7e is therefore the examination of our ward philosophy as compared to that of the Burford unit.

The current ward philosophy originates from 1990 when the ward team were gathered together for development work when the ward was

This is a statement of some of our shared values and beliefs that guide our nursing practice on 7e.

Every patient deserves the unconditional warm regard of the nurses. Every person is a unique individual with social, psychological, spiritual and physical needs who should be allowed to make informed choices which the nurses will respect. If it seems appropriate the nurses will encourage family and friends to be closely involved in the patient's care.

To us, the most important aspect of nursing is caring. This includes the development of a partnership between the nurse and the patient. The aim of the partnership is to meet the patient's needs but at the same time foster personal control and the growth of independence.

Nursing care is provided by a team of nurses each with a unique and valuable contribution to make. We acknowledge the importance of continuity of care and endeavour to provide this for our patients by using a primary nursing system. On admission every patient is assigned to a small team of nurses, one of whom will be the named primary nurse. This primary nurse will be responsible for the planning of care with the patient using a systematic approach.

Whenever on duty the primary nurse will look after the patient. In her/his absence the associate nurse(s) will continue care as planned. Any unqualified member of staff will be supervised by a qualified member of the ward team.

Knowledge enables people to look after themselves and helps prevent reoccurrence or exacerbation of illness. It is therefore an important nursing responsibility to educate patients and their families.

Nurses are part of a multidisciplinary team which works together for the benefit of patients. Success of this team depends on cooperation and good communication.

Nursing care is prescribed using up-to-date nursing knowledge and in the light of experience. It is every nurse's responsibility to continue her/his education and share this knowledge with others. Learning opportunities are provided on the ward and staff are encouraged to attend study days whenever possible.

Fig. 7.2   7e ward philosophy (*circa* 1990).

being decorated. Only four members (out of about twenty) survive from that time. The need for change to reflect different influences and personnel (Johns, 1990) has therefore perhaps not been met. However, the philosophy has been discussed on two occasions since 1990 and agreed to be adequate by the majority of the ward team. There are possibly questions to be asked about this apparent adequacy. For example:

- Is the philosophy still an integral part of people's thinking?
- Is the notion of a ward philosophy perceived as relevant to practice or is it seen as a paper exercise?
- Is it seen as a subject worth spending time and energy on?

The current philosophy (Fig. 7.2) is analyzed here using the key components of a philosophy identified by Johns (1989):

- External environment of care
- Internal environment of care
- Social viability
- The nature of care.

External environment of care

The external environment of care is described as relating to the context and function of nursing practice in a given area. At present, notions of environmental factors which enable as well as constrain the provision of nursing care are not contained within the philosophy. However, there are factors within the external environment which have a bearing on the care provided on the ward. Recognition of such factors is important if the philosophy is to be used as a document which:

> '... attempts to capture the tension between the reality of practice and the beliefs and values of practitioners.' (Johns 1991)

Such a function renders the philosophy a relevant source for the generation of statements concerning the outcomes of nursing on the ward. Since a development of clinically-relevant quality measures is also part of the NDU remit of the ward, it becomes doubly important that the philosophy of the ward is relevant to practice at the present time.

Nursing leadership in Oxfordshire has pioneered a model of professional nursing which is designed to potentiate nurses as autonomous professionals in their dealings with patients. An environment exists where nurses make decisions about the work that they will undertake within clear guidelines. Nurses are encouraged to take maximum individual responsibility according to professional judgement based on the following guidance:

- The individual nurses are responsible and accountable for their own decisions and actions.
- They must be able to defend those decisions and actions as being in the best interest of their patients.
- They must only undertake work for which they are trained and are competent to perform.

These guidelines from the Oxford District Health Authority Guidelines for Nursing Practice (Pembrey 1989) bear close resemblance to the United Kingdom Central Council's latest edition of Code of Professional Conduct (1992).

Environmental constraints are most apparent in considering the statements (see Fig. 7.2) concerning the manner in which care delivery is organized. For example:

> 'We acknowledge the importance of continuity of care and endeavour to provide this for our patients by using a primary nursing system. On admission every patient is assigned to a small team of nurses, one of whom will be the named primary nurse.

However, this does not always happen. The continuity demanded by this statement requires a degree of organizational complexity, which with the demands placed by annual leave, days off and study days becomes difficult to the extent where continuity cannot always be afforded. This difficulty is compounded by the high turnover of patients on the ward. In effect this means that many of the people that nurses meet stay for between 24 and 48 hours. Some stay for a number of weeks or even months. As a result, the approaches nurses utilize conceptually and in their records need to be flexible to meet widely varying paces of work.

The opinions of the ward team elicited so far would indicate that at present this is not necessarily the case. The number of comments concerning how much time is consumed in recording assessments and care plans for patients would seem to indicate, along with the patchy nature of records found in patients' files, that the means of satisfactorily representing nursing thoughts and actions have not yet been found. This applies particularly to patients who stay in hospital for relatively short periods. The pressures placed on the continuity of care by the members of the nursing team put great demands on their skills of communication. Arguably, such a degree of task complexity requires clarity when it comes to outlining the responsibilities of nurses both individually and collectively. At present this clarity could be said to be lacking from the statement (see Fig. 7.2):

> 'This primary nurse will be responsible for the planning of care ... using a systematic approach.'

Especially so in the light of team members holding differing views as to the merits and content of such a systematic approach.

The Oxford Radcliffe Hospital provides emergency services for a wide geographical area. It works with a network of more specialized centres and a number of community hospitals. Nurses within the hospital can expect to work within a complex web of other professionals both within and outside the hospital. To name but a few, this web can potentially include:

- doctors (physicians, specialists to whom patients are referred, general practitioners)
- other nurses (district nurses, nurses in other units and hospitals, practice nurses)
- physiotherapists
- occupational therapists
- dietitians
- speech therapists
- social workers
- ambulance service personnel
- radiographers
- electrocardiograph technicians.

The medical wards at the Oxford Radcliffe Hospital fulfil a number of functions, some or all of which may be carried out in providing nursing to an individual. These can include:

- the assessment and support of the acutely ill person
- complementing and supporting medical intervention
- the initiation and provision of rehabilitation
- discharge planning
- health education
- the provision of palliative care when a person is dying.

Given the broad range of possible activities that can notionally be undertaken, any philosophical underpinnings need to support a broad range of approaches to working which are responsive to the needs of both long and short stay patients who are encountering a wide range of problems. Such flexibility would need to be represented by any model adopted. The practical application of the model would need to be easily learnt, easily used both for record keeping and as a tool to enable the understanding and analysis of patients' experience and be able to facilitate varied degrees of use.

The 7e ward philosophy could be developed more in relation to exploring the tensions between practical constraints and the ideological aspirations of the ward team. At present the philosophy focuses principally on the nurse–patient relationship while acknowledging the potential for involvement of family and friends in a patient's care. The ward's status as an NDU places new responsibilities on it and these have yet to be expressed explicitly within the ward's philosophy. Such responsibilities are apparent in the Burford philosophy and the resultant model for practice. A fuller consideration of contextual issues related to the ward's position and function both within and outside the Oxford

Radcliffe Hospital in future reformulation of the philosophy may help team members situate their work within a broader picture.

Internal environment

The internal environment is concerned with issues such as relationships between nurses and other health professionals. The Burford philosophy (Johns 1991) as well as Johns' work on therapeutic teams (1992) describe the need for the relationships between staff to be founded on similar humanistic principles to those between nurse and patient. The idea that nurses cannot convey the acceptance and warmth that they aspire to without providing each other with similar support is contained within our philosophy to a certain extent. The lived experience of working in the ward suggests that nurses adopt similar attitudes to each other as they do to patients, if anecdotal comments of those who come to work on the ward are to be believed.

Similar support systems to those described at Burford are well established. Regular review of performance takes place, albeit informally at times. Regular meetings are held to discuss ward progress. Various forms of personal and professional development are actively encouraged and supported through an agreed minimum of study leave per year. The devising and refinement of flexible work patterns has been defined and is under constant revision so that team members may optimize their contribution to the ward as a whole while following other paths in their lives (for instance, having a family or becoming a full-time student).

The organization of the ward's nursing team reflects beliefs influenced by devolvement of responsibility. The work on supportive hierarchies (Ryan, 1989) has been influential. A support hierarchy has as its objective quality care for its clients wherein control of events is ideally vested in the client. The provider of the service (the practitioner) is accountable to the client and is supported by senior colleagues who act as resources and facilitators, as well as educators, associates, learners and ancillary staff. The practitioner works in collaboration with other members of the multi-disciplinary team. In effect, the pyramidal nature of a hierarchy, with leaders on top and workers as the base, is turned on its head. The resources of the organization are employed to support the practitioners in their encounters with clients.

On 7e, a system of collective decision-making has evolved. The ward is led by a group of senior practitioners who support the team as a whole. Administrative tasks which were traditionally the domain of the ward sister are devolved throughout the team and rotated on a regular basis.

It can be said therefore that in terms of what happens on the ward there is a strong relationship between the nature of nurse–patient relationships and those between the nurses themselves. Relationships are orientated towards affording development of, and opportunity for, individual responsibility.

May (1992), in a qualitative study involving the observation of 22 staff nurses in Scotland, speaks of patients being given 'multiple and disconnected identities' by the various staff that they encounter during a hospital stay. In a busy teaching hospital such as the Oxford Radcliffe the majority of occupational groups involved in day-to-day care of patients are subject to relatively high turnover. House officers may work on a ward for between two and six months, senior house officers only slightly longer. Physiotherapists, dietitians and occupational therapists move every four months. The constancy is provided by nurses who usually work for at least a year if not considerably longer in one place.

Speaking from the perspective of a nurse who has seen medical and paramedical staff pass through my own clinical area, the notion of patients being given 'multiple and disconnected identities' is persuasive. Conflict may occasionally result. While such conflicts may be productively resolved through negotiation, a situation where there is a consistent and unified multidisciplinary approach for any length of time is difficult to achieve. The articulation of nursing philosophy is a recent phenomenon and seems to have a unifying influence on nursing staff when they have been involved in its writing. The author of this chapter carried out a small scale grounded theory study of five registered nurses working in primary nursing settings. A contextual factor underlying the way in which informants worked was identified by them as being the ward philosophy.

However, there remains potential for philosophical statements of intent to be used as one means of communicating the beliefs and intentions of the most stable work group in most hospital settings. Anecdotally it seems that nurses on 7e believe that they use a similar approach in their dealings with patients. This seems to help in underpinning the role of patient advocate. Nonetheless, the extent to which this approach is clear to others within the multidisciplinary group is uncertain.

The ward philosophy is used as part of new staff members' introduction to the ward. It has also been illustrated in a photograph album for patients. Neither of these initiatives have been formally evaluated, although they seem to be valued. It seems, however, that as a statement of group intent, the full power of the philosophy has yet to be explored on the ward.

Social viability

As described by Johns (1991), the concept of social viability is adopted from the work of Dorothy Johnson (1974). Three criteria were suggested which may be helpful in evaluating a model for nursing.

(1) Social congruence is based on the extent to which decisions and actions fulfil social expectations.
(2) Social significance is determined by the extent to which actions based on a model make a difference to patient outcomes.
(3) Social utility is determined by examining the extent to which clear direction for practice education and research is provided.

While, arguably, it is as yet incomplete, the 7e ward philosophy enjoys a degree of social significance. Its content is shared with patients on the ward, usually at an early stage of their stay. Within environments where public expectations are to 'toe the line' when in hospital (Waterworth & Luker 1990), notions of active participation in their own care may frequently seem alien to patients. With support from their nurses, however, patients can journey from feeling that they have to conform to a set of expectations to a point where they can express themselves more freely. This is an area of the ward philosophy which can possibly be evaluated. Others are less easily determined. For instance, the notion of 'unconditional warm regard'.

Political statements are implicit within the 7e philosophy; in particular, the belief that in an acute setting patients deserve the care of a professional nurse. This belief is underpinned by the beliefs of nursing leaders such as Pembrey (1984) and by more recent work examining the relative merits of differing skill and grade mixes. Work on skill mix has examined the value-for-money of care delivered by qualified nurses (Hancock 1992). She cites studies such as that by Helt and Jellinek (1988) in arguing that a high ratio of qualified nurses has the potential to increase efficiency. The study '*Ward Nursing Quality and Grade Mix*' (Bagust *et al.* 1992) has suggested that in some settings a smaller work force with a higher proportion of qualified nurses delivers higher quality patient care and is more cost effective.

The nature of care

According to the 7e philosophy, caring is the most important aspect of nursing. Although the exact nature of caring is not articulated further within the context of the 7e ward philosophy, there are components of caring that are implicit within the philosophy. These include:

- The development of a partnership between nurse and patient with the partnership orientated towards both meeting the person's needs while fostering personal control and growth.
- The provision of knowledge to avoid future reoccurrence or exacerbation of illness.

Stress is laid on the importance of the use of up-to-date knowledge as well as experience in the prescription of nursing care.

The influence of those concepts from within humanism and phenomenology described in Johns (1991) are apparent; in particular, the notion of working with patients towards their improved health through considering social, psychological, physical and spiritual needs.

Given that the Burford model of nursing flows from philosophical concepts, it is a necessary first step to examine the congruity between those concepts and the philosophy adopted on 7e in considering the suitability of the model for adaptation to an acute medical setting. The external environment of the two units is different to an extent. The difference lies in the great complexity of relationships and speed of turnover on 7e. Nurses on 7e possibly meet patients at a different stage of their hospital career than at Burford. The internal environment is more explicitly examined within the Burford philosophy; however, initiatives on 7e exemplify staff relationships which parallel those we strive to offer patients.

The principal areas of congruence between the two philosophies are in dealing with nurse–patient and nurse–nurse relationships. An area of divergence is that of a more individualistic approach described within the 7e philosophy than that found within the Burford philosophy. However, the degree of divergence in practice is difficult to assess. Overall it would seem that the philosophical approaches off both units have much in common and that the model arising from the Burford philosophy may be congruent with practice on 7e.

Using the BNDU model

Pragmatism

Since reading Johns (1991) I have used ideas contained within the model in my practice. Similarly, colleagues have tried out the assessment strategy in particular. The immediate appeal of the model lies in the posing of the very simple and pragmatic question, 'What information do I need to nurse this patient?' It is this pragmatic approach that we frequently adopt as a response to an environment where the demands of workload fluctuate rapidly. As a result, the priorities in our work are primarily those of providing care and time required for completing nursing records is resented, especially where its content is perceived to be repetitive and irrelevant. Of twelve respondents to a questionnaire that I asked my colleagues to complete, eight identified paperwork as the most unpopular aspect of the nursing process. Six respondents also identified present practice as repetitive, for example:

'Do we really need to write at such lengths that which is of no relevance to us and which creates no problem or is of little or no relevance?'

The responses to the questionnaire support findings of a detailed qualitative study of four Canadian nurses (Howse & Bailey 1992). The authors describe what they call intrinsic and extrinsic factors which make documentation difficult for nurses. Intrinsic factors include difficulties with written expression and the feeling that 'doing it is more important than writing it'. Extrinsic factors include the format of documents and the time required to complete them within busy and pressured work settings.

In the course of keeping in mind the strategy of the BNDU model while working with patients, I have found that it lends itself to flexible approaches of documenting issues of concern to colleagues. For example, the accepted practice of waiting for a relationship to form with a patient before formal assessment can mean that the amount of information available about patients can be small. Some of the ward team have adopted the practice of presenting an abbreviated sketch of the most prominent concerns about a patient to 'fill the gap' before a fuller assessment is presented. At times, this sketch can suffice for a patient whose stay is short or relatively uncomplicated.

For example, this summary was written about a middle-aged woman, Susan, when she was admitted with suspected pulmonary embolus:

Areas of concern

- Married woman who has been unwell for 5 days, 'bad chest'.
- Pain, worse on inspiration, left lower chest, mainly at back.
- Productive cough with blood stained sputum.
- ? pulmonary embolus, no apparent risk factors.

While this summary could undoubtedly have been fuller, and as this person's time in hospital went on, more complex areas of concern became apparent, it provided an answer to an immediate question of, 'What information do I need to nurse this patient?' From this base I could then, equally briefly, identify, 'How can I help this person?', framing both her and her family's concerns – fear, uncertainty and pain – with those which arose from my own knowledge – safety and accurate diagnosis. Using such an economic approach, the cue, 'How can I help this person?' summarizes the assessment in terms of a plan of care, the timescale of which can be specified:

Plan for the first 24 hours

- Give analgesia as prescribed, ask Susan how well it's working.
- Susan wants to know what is happening!
- Ask Susan to stay on her bed until diagnosis is confirmed (or not).
- Measure her and provide her with anti-embolism stockings.
- IV cannula in left hand inserted on admission, monitor anti-coagulant therapy.
- Observations as specified on chart.

With a more complex situation the BNDU model strategy seems to help the nurse identify issues that are relevant to patients, their families and other nurses. Not that this is a unique attribute. Other models that I have used (Orem; Roper *et al.*, Roy & Andrews) facilitate problem identification; that is, after all, part of the intention! However, where this particular strategy is different for me is in the sense of the narrative arising from the dialogue.

For example, consider the initial assessment of Ted; a case study:

Ted is in his sixties. Recently retired from working as a storesman. He was once a miner. He lives with his wife and has a daughter who lives nearby. He sees her often. He came to the ward two days ago after becoming increasingly ill over the last month. He finds swallowing difficult. He gets breathless easily, but he can still care for himself. We do not know as yet why Ted has these symptoms. He has already been investigated for possible cancer. He says that he is most concerned just to know one way or another what is going on. He agrees that he is apprehensive; he says that he is taking it 'day to day'. He has lost weight (about half-a-stone over six weeks). His wife and daughter seem to understand the situation in much the same way as Ted.

This narrative clearly indicated issues of concern to the person involved. In this case they were partly to do with psychological aspects – uncertainty and fear – and partly to do with physical problems – weight loss and breathlessness. The assessment arose out of several conversations with ideas being checked out with Ted. These conversations enabled me to focus and refocus care on what was concerning Ted most. Conceptual models usually feature an assessment structure. Implementation of a model has often featured dedicated documentation. Nurses that I have observed and worked with have a tendency to subvert such external structures, finding them restrictive and inhibiting (R. Garbett, unpublished observations). While the variety and originality that is manifest is invigorating, such a situation is unsatisfactory from the point of view of the need for a team of people working in concert to have a degree of congruency in the way that they work. There is also a need to consider the visitors to the ward: nursing students, bank and agency nurses, and nurses visiting the nursing development unit from outside.

The intention of the assessment strategy being used to elicit a patient's 'situated meaning' (Benner & Wrubel 1989) is explicit (Johns 1991). That the strategy enables this to be articulated is as much to do with the nurses using it, but the process seems to be aided by the use of cues rather than the presentation of a structure into which the nurses try to fit what they have learnt. With use and adaptation the initial pragmatism of an approach which allows for a variety of approaches to recording and presenting information within an identifiable strategy has the potential to unify practice without constraining it.

Telling a story

> 'In the telling of a story from practice, nursing knowledge is preserved in its wholeness; understanding is enhanced.' (Arndt 1992, p.287)

Using the BNDU strategy seems to help the telling of a patient's story, preserving its relevance to them while indicating priorities for the nurse. When collecting my observations, conversations and interpretations, as well as those of others, into a nursing assessment using a more structured approach, the use of headings can prove restrictive. A person's experience does not lend itself easily to categorization, especially at the end of a long and busy day (the questionnaires that my colleagues completed suggest that despite their best intentions this is still the time of day when nursing notes are completed). While, as academic exercises, I have found the use of Orem's Self Care Deficit model (1991) or Roy's Stress Adaptation theory (Roy & Andrews 1991) useful and illuminating analytical tools, my experience of using them in practice is less fruitful. The notions underlying them are easily diluted by demands on time and thought, even when their concepts are familiar to me. The points concerning the difficulty of complex concepts and language are discussed elsewhere in this chapter.

The example given in the initial assessment of Ted (above) shows how a narrative that is relevant to the patient's situation can arise without the need for an external structure. Writing more or less 'from the hip' was also much quicker than attempting to fit information under headings.

The counter argument that may be posed is that the above assessment leaves out a lot of information (indeed, for purposes of anonymity it is abbreviated). Here Hall's (1964) point is instructive: 'We can only nurse what the patient allows us to nurse'. After two shifts of spending short periods of working together, this is what Ted had shared with me. I had tried to avoid replicating questions that doctors would have already asked him other than checking points from his medical notes that I was unsure about. My intention was to produce a starting point that was relevant, brief and from where I could plan safe and appropriate care. The reader must take my word that this was indeed the case.

Ted's assessment written here seems hollow in comparison with the scribbled side of A4 paper which I sat and discussed with a very scared but brave man. For him and for me, at least, the words are charged with the emotion of a vital passage in his life and the lives of his family. The bare words contain the pride that was evident when he spoke of his origins in the north of England, the disappointment at becoming ill so soon after retirement, and the resignation to the possibility that he may be gravely ill. His validation of my efforts reassured me that I was directing my energies appropriately. That is not to say that the priorities for care were all Ted's, but using the BNDU strategy seemed to help me find the unity between his agenda and my own and see the inter-relatedness of his problems.

Some practical points

A model for nursing can be perceived as more of a paper exercise than a practical one. My experience of using the BNDU model is that it lends itself to transcending such problems. Using its strategy does not seem to hamper me and it can be applied flexibly to the production of written communications for patients and colleagues. The intention for nursing assessments on the ward is that they should be living documents which can be added to. From the nursing process questionnaires it would also seem that there is a body of opinion which indicates an aspiration amongst the nursing team for members of the multidisciplinary team to consult nursing notes. A barrier to this which has been identified is the difficulty in accessing information within nursing notes in their current format. Accordingly, it may be useful for additions to the assessment, after the initial narrative account, to be given some sort of heading to indicate what the new information is about, for example, *social situation* or *appetite*.

Johns (1991) in describing the model, places most emphasis on the cue questions for assessment. The care planning aspect of nursing process, he suggests, lends itself most readily to addressing physical problems. While I would tentatively agree, it is suggested here that the formulation of care plans and their content in using the model requires more consideration. The precise function of the care plan is a vexed question:

> 'No other single issue, thought, technique, problem or phenomenon has received as much attention, has been as much taught, talked about, worked at, read about and cried over with so little success. No other issue in nursing has caused so much guilt and energy to be misspent. Yet no other piece of paper in a hospital is as devoid of information as that entitled nursing care plan.' (Manthey 1980)

A variety of functions are expected from nursing notes in general: communication, accountability and auditability, for example. The volume and detail of records required for the above purposes can prove problematic (de la Cuesta 1983; Reed, unpublished observations; Porter 1990; Howse & Bailey 1992). De la Cuesta's informants saw care plans as 'imposed formalities'. Reed's doctoral work describes how, where the format of nursing documentation is imposed by managers, the relevance of nursing records for nurses themselves is not apparent. Porter, in examining power relations between nurses and doctors, observed that 'the lack of utility value of the nursing process in comparison with the labour required ... has led to disillusionment.' Howse and Bailey noted persistent antipathy towards documentation generally, both in their review of literature and in their case study of four Canadian nurses, this antipathy being brought about by inflexible and prescriptive formats as well as lack of confidence and skills in written expression.

There is apparently no clear and unified picture of what nursing records are for. The summary of findings for the Department of Health's investigation (1992) defines the purpose of records vaguely, reporting a need to underpin 'good care' with records. A lack of understanding among nurses of the status of records and their retrospective use as legal evidence is reported. It was also noted that systems of care organization (primary and team nursing) where the patients are better known to nurses resulted in 'less recorded information'. In the same paper the recommendations include the specification of information needed in nursing records in order to use them for workload calculation, as well as the need for service purchasers to specify 'the required standards of nursing records'.

With such uncertainty about the precise function of nursing records it is difficult to plan developments with any accuracy. It is safe to say, however, that extrinsic factors may impinge. For instance, in Oxford-shire the implementation of the Care in the Community Act has resulted in the hasty introduction of a standardized discharge planning package, the explicit reason for the standardized format being ease of audit.

Problems of definition on a large scale do not seem to advance nurses far with the situated question of what nursing records should or should not contain. Johns (1991) suggests care plans should be about physical needs with some form of 'professional notes' of their work with patients for use in communication between primary and associate nurses. The nursing team on 7e seem to adapt traditional modes of care planning to varying needs. Where care is self evident then this fact is recorded on the plan, for example, 'The usual care for someone with a urinary catheter, except...'

Where a patient's problem does not lend itself to a concrete goal, then a goal may not be included in the plan, for example, where the problem is psycho-social in nature and not easily reduced to the reductionistic nature of a care plan. It may be that a particular area of concern is not yet fully understood and that the care plan is used as a focus for gathering information in order to then formulate a plan. This approach was used when it was unclear how much potential a person who had suffered an extensive cerebrovascular accident had for rehabilitation, the goal being to describe the person's behaviour to facilitate assessment.

It may be that an important component of developing practice is to ask similarly pragmatic questions to those contained within the BNDU model: what sort of information do we need to communicate to each other and how do we present it? Experience suggests that the nurses' judgement as to how busy they are and what sort of continuity of care is available to a patient or group of patients to an extent dictates the amount of detail contained in, and the manner of presentation of, nursing records.

It may be that a repertoire of methods and approaches is employed which reflects the varying needs of patients and changeable pace of work on the ward. Given a consensus amongst the ward team, a regular review process and a means by which new members of the team can be orientated to modes of practice, such an approach could conceivably suffice to ensure a consistent approach from the point of view of communication. Catering for the needs of auditability and accountability is perhaps more problematic since they are essentially outside any single ward's control.

Consideration of the cue questions

In this section I will examine the kinds of information which the cue questions helped me to gather. While the cue questions are not headings but guides to answering the core question of 'What information do I need to be able to nurse this person?', experience of utilizing the cues in practice leads me to suggest some adaptations. These adaptations take the form of additional cues and amplifications of the present cues. The purpose of suggesting additional cues is twofold: firstly, it is to aid my own understanding of the information I need to care for a patient in my own setting, and secondly, it is to help the communication of this understanding to colleagues.

'Who is this person?'

Johns (1991) suggests that this question leads the nurse to consider the person within the context of their social and cultural world. The information which may therefore be gathered includes the roles a person performs in their life as a baseline against which the effects of their present situation can be assessed.

At times it has proved relevant to include the perceptions of a patient's 'significant others'; indeed a holistic standpoint requires that these perspectives be taken into account. Various disease processes as well as the stress of ill-health affect a person's perception of themselves. Such an effect may be organic, as in neurological conditions or where biochemical disturbances are taking place, or psychological. Whatever the cause the perceptions of a person's family and friends lend breadth to an understanding of what has happened to a person as a result of ill-health. In an area such as a general medical ward where many patients are experiencing multiple pathologies the information provided by those who know the patient can be vital in unravelling what is happening. Presented only with the behaviour of an acutely ill person without the information available from others who know them can lead to distorted perceptions on the part of health professionals. Two examples from my own practice come to mind.

The first example concerns a man who had suffered severe neurological damage. As a result, nursing him could present certain practical difficulties if he became uncooperative or even aggressive. Understanding from his family that the way he behaved represented an accentuation of how he usually responded to being told what to do helped us to be more patient in our approach to providing him with essential care.

The second example concerns an episode where the lack of corroborating information about a person made understanding what was happening to him difficult. A middle-aged man was admitted to the ward with signs and behaviour consistent with hyperglycaemia and acute infection. He was confused, irritable and uncooperative. What was not known was that he also had a psychiatric condition. Given that he had no immediate family and friends with him at the time of admission it took a matter of days to gather enough information to understand what was happening to him.

'What health event brings this person into hospital?'

Given the holistic basis of the model, it is important to blend together perspectives on the health event underlying a patient's contact with health care. A medical diagnosis is just one part of this. From the point of view of a nurse trying to construct, with a patient, a picture of their present health event it is important to find out what they have been experiencing and how they understand it. Such information is necessary for the nursing function of health education and promotion.

The importance of reaching mutual understandings with patients rather than adopting a blanket approach to health education was illustrated when a middle-aged woman was admitted to the ward from the Coronary Care Unit. She had been given both written and verbal information about what had happened, about the effect it would have on her and so on, but it was clear that little had sunk in so far. On talking to her about her understanding of her illness she admitted that she knew very little about the workings of the body and did not really understand the explanations given to her. As a result I tried using diagrams and drawings in an overall approach that avoided giving too much information at once.

'How must this person be feeling?'

The root of this question is identified as being the notion of 'situated meaning' (Benner & Wrubel 1989). It is described as a broad question that covers both the patient and their family and as relating not only to the main reason for admission but also to other concerns that may need attending to. For me, paying attention to how the patient is feeling also highlights the dynamic nature of the notion of assessment. The adoption and internalization by a nurse of a central theme – 'What information do I need to be able to nurse this person?' – aided by a series of cue questions helps focus the cognitive activities which practising nurses may be constantly engaged in.

While assessment information is mainly a matter of establishing matters of concern to which nurses need to address themselves it is also an ongoing activity (R. Garbett, unpublished observations). De la Cuesta (1983) made the observation that the nursing process, in UK use at least, loses its dynamic nature with feedback loops between the various stages and becomes a linear rather than cyclical model. The Burford model's fluid structure seems to lend itself to being an internal tool that can be employed to make sense of ever-changing situations. A patient's experience of a hospital stay is complex. Their emotional responses are likewise complex and require of the nurse reflexivity and the ability to adapt quickly to a person's changing moods and responses.

'How has this event affected usual life patterns and roles?'

Consideration of this question is, as Johns (1991) states, important in setting appropriate goals against a picture of what is normal for a particular person. In essence, this is an 'activities of living' question and would lend itself to the adaptation of various classifications apart from Roper *et al.*'s. This question also has considerable diagnostic power. Increasingly within general hospitals there is an emphasis on expediting discharge or referral of patients as soon as is appropriate. A patient's abilities with regard to activities of living are important in planning for discharge or transfer to other settings (rehabilitation centres, community hospitals, nursing homes, home with social service support, and so on). Within the acute setting it may also be that referral is required to other members of the multidisciplinary team to provide assistance in some way (physiotherapy, occupational therapy, social work, and so on). In identifying areas of concern the nurse can also identify the degree of permanence of the changes in life patterns and roles, for instance, how long before someone who has had a heart attack can start driving, going out or resume a sexual relationship.

'How does this person make me feel?'

The intention of this question shares common ground with the notion of 'bracketing' in phenomenological research (Morse 1991) – phenomenologists describe dealing with their own biases by 'bracketing out' their prejudgments and commitments so as to see new phenomena clearly (Cohen 1987) – and with notions of 'emotional competence' in the literature on counselling where practitioners' own concerns do not 'drive or distort' the care that they give (Heron 1990).

The inclusion of such a question under the heading of assessment cue is innovative. Emotional reactions of all kinds may influence nurses' delivery of care or the equity of care that they deliver to a group of people. This question epitomizes for me the model's utility as a tool to be used in approaching interactions with patients rather than simply as a template for the nursing process. In fact, explicitly recording information about one's feelings about a patient may well be rare in an acute medical setting. However, considerations of emotional reactions to a patient and their situation will influence handovers, interdisciplinary communication, and so on. Attempting to reflect upon feelings about a patient also provides grounds for comparison with the ideas contained within the ward philosophy.

'How can I help this person?'

The notions underlying this and the following question lend themselves to that part of assessment which is diagnostic in nature (Leddy & Pepper 1989). The question represents a drawing together of the information that the nurse has gathered and interpreted. This information is then used to identify strategies for nursing interventions which can be offered to the patient and/or their family.

It may be that for future use with some form of information management system this cue question can be linked with a framework of nursing diagnosis. Present taxonomies that are available have been developed in the USA and presently could be argued to be conceptually and linguistically unsuitable for adoption in the UK. However, given the widespread introduction of computer systems in the UK, it may be wise to consider how approaches to data gathering such as that represented by the Burford holistic model can be adapted to allow their use.

'What is important for this person to make their stay in hospital comfortable?'

Including a diagnostic question that is framed from the patient's point of view encourages the nurse to move away from the dilemma posed in previous discussions about nursing process, that of to whose problems is nursing being addressed (de la Cuesta 1983)? This and the above question encourage the nurse to reflect on any discrepancies there might be between their perspective and that of the patient. Thinking about how the patient may be helped is only part of the task, a task completed by exploring what the patient wants. This is far from being a simple task and the components of the debates about the nature of nurse–patient relationships are to be found elsewhere (for example, Gadow 1985 amongst many others).

'What support does this person have in life?'

In an acute medical setting where the emphasis is increasingly on swift turnover of patients, (at present the average stay in medical beds in the Oxford Radcliffe is about five days), the need to address issues concerning the support a patient has in their community is of primary importance. It is therefore a question which needs to be asked as early as possible after admission; indeed, with the implementation of the Care in the Community Act it is a requirement to 'screen' new admissions to ascertain whether support will be needed after discharge. Separate documentation has been introduced in Oxford in an attempt to standardize the kinds of information gathered about the support available to a patient. For the purposes of learning to employ the model it may be that for some areas at least this question is better situated higher in the list of cue questions.

Given the holistic basis of the model, questions of this nature require the nurse to broaden their focus in looking at issues of care after discharge from a variety of points of view. For instance, while a patient's daughter may want to look after a disabled parent at home, it may be necessary to encourage her to explore the needs of her own family as well as her own knowledge and skills before final arrangements for discharge are made. This question may benefit from including a sense of what further support is needed.

'How do they view the future for themselves and others?'

As Johns (1991) observes, exploration of this question often requires a trusting relationship for patients to expose what their concerns for the future are. Moreover, responses to health crises may be characterized by inaccurate expectations about future problems or abilities. Exploring how the patient and those around them see the future can help set the agenda for the provision of information and referral to other agencies. In the case of Ted above, he anticipated becoming weaker and having more pain, and his wife anticipated not being able to cope looking after him. The measures that we took included initiating alterations in their home, making contact with the local hospice services and district nursing, and establishing an effective drug regime with Ted learning how some of the drugs worked so that he could tailor them to his needs.

It may be that a useful additional question may be, 'What information does this person need?' In the same way as the questions 'How can I help this person?' and 'What is important for this person to make their stay in hospital comfortable?' have a diagnostic element to them, posing the question 'What information does this person need?' would, along with the addition suggested to the question 'What further support is needed?', have a similarly diagnostic function. These additional cues may facilitate the planning of strategies for health promotion and community support on discharge.

Classification of the cue questions

Using the cue questions to guide my information-gathering has led me to loosely classify them as follows:

Baseline questions
- 'Who is this person?'
- 'What health event brings this person into hospital?'
- 'What support does this person have in life?'
- ('How does this person make me feel?')

Questions identifying areas of concern
- 'How must this person be feeling?'
- 'How has this event affected usual life patterns and roles (activities of living)?'
- 'What support does this person have in life?'
- 'How do they view the future for themselves and others?'
- ('How does this person make me feel?')

Diagnostic questions
- 'How can I help this person?'
- 'What is important for this person to make their stay in hospital comfortable?'
- 'What additional support might they need?'
- 'What information does this person need?'
- ('How does this person make me feel?')

The changing pace and complexity of hospital work, as well as the reflexive approach taken towards individual situations, means that any classification must be flexible. In terms of acute care I have found that the above grouping of the questions helps focus my efforts in a way that reflects the patient's care setting career. An attempt at classification is not so much an attempt to guide the gathering of information; rather it is an attempt to help order it. The question 'How does this person make me feel?' is included at each stage because of its potential for affording perspective on how the nurse is working. It is put in parentheses to denote that thoughts arising from the question are unlikely to be included in permanent records.

Conclusions

As I stated at the outset of this chapter, this is an account of a journey that is ongoing. My discussion is of early experiences with using the

BNDU model and is far from exhaustive. In the first part of the chapter I concluded that there exists a degree of congruence between the philosophical beliefs of nurses at Burford Community Hospital and the nurses on my own ward in an acute medical unit, on the basis of which it is considered to be worthwhile exploring the use of the model in practice. Some of the practical points discovered so far are discussed. For me, the main power of the model lies in its deceptive simplicity. It is at once pragmatic and profound, useful both as an aid to articulating information about a patient and as a framework to guide the building of a relationship between nurse and patient through which both can learn and grow.

References

Arndt, M.J. (1992) Caring as everydayness. *Journal of Holistic Nursing*, **10**(4), 285–93.

Bagust, A., Slack, R. & Oakley, J. (1992) *Ward Nursing Quality and Grade Mix.* York Health Economics Consortium, University of York.

Benner, P. & Wrubel, J. (1989) *The Primacy of Caring: Stress and coping in health and illness.* Addison–Wesley Publishing Company, Menlo Park, California.

Champion, R. (1992) The philosophy of an honours degree programme in nursing and midwifery. In *Developing Professional Education*, (eds H. Bines & D. Watson). Open University Press, Milton Keynes.

Chapman, P. (1990) A critical perspective. In *Models for Nursing 2*, (eds B. Kershaw & J. Salvage). Scutari Press, Harrow, Middlesex.

Chinn, P.L. & Jacobs, M.K. (1983) *Theory and Nursing: A Systematic Approach*, 2nd edn. C.V. Mosby, St. Louis.

Clarke, M. (1986) Action and reflection: practice and theory in nursing. *Journal of Advanced Nursing*, **11**(1) 3–11.

Cohen, M.S. (1987) An historical overview of the phenomenological movement. *Image: The Journal of Nursing Scholarship*, **19**(1), 31–34.

de la Cuesta (1983) The nursing process from development to implementation. *Journal of Advanced Nursing*, **8**, 365–71.

Department of Health (1992) *Summary of report of nursing records study: good practice* (PL/CNO (92) 10) HMSO, London.

Draper, P. (1990) The development of theory in British nursing: current position and future prospects. *Journal of Advanced Nursing*, **15**(1), 12–15.

Gadow, S. (1985) Nurse and patient: the caring relationship. In *Caring, Curing, Coping*, (eds A.H. Bishop & J.R. Scudder). University of Alabama Press, Birmingham, Alabama.

Garbett, R. (1993) Lecturer practitioners in Oxford: addressing the challenge of the theory practice gap. In: *Nursing: Care in Crisis*, (eds G. Bryckyzsnka & M. Jolley). C.V. Mosby, London.

Gordon, D. (1984) Research application: identifying the use and misuse of formal models in nursing practice. In *From Novice to Expert: Excellence and Power in Nursing*, (ed. P. Benner). Addison–Wesley Publishing Company, Menlo Park, California.

Greenwood, J. (1984) Nursing Research: a position paper. *Journal of Advanced Nursing*, **9**(1), 77–82.

Gruending, D. (1985) Nursing theory: a vehicle for professionalisation? *Journal of Advanced Nursing*, **10**(6), 553–8.

Hall, L.E. (1964) Nursing – What is it? *The Canadian Nurse*, **60**(2), 150–54.

Hancock, C. (1992) *Nurses and skill mix: what are the issues?* Paper presented at the Nurses Skill Mix conference, St Bartholomews Hospital, London.

Helt, E., Jelinek, R.C. (1988) In the wake of cost cutting, nursing productivity and quality improve. *Nursing Management*, **19**(6), 36–48.

Heron, J. (1990) *Helping the Client*. Sage Publications, London.

Howse, E. & Bailey, J. (1992) Resistance to documentation – a nursing research issue. *International Journal of Nursing Studies*, **29**(4), 371–80.

Johns, C.C. (1989) Developing a philosophy for practice: Part 1. *Nursing Practice*, **3**(1), 2–5.

Johns, C.C. (1990) Developing a philosophy for practice: Part 2. *Nursing Practice*, **3**(2), 2–5.

Johns, C.C. (1991) The Burford Nursing Developing Unit holistic model of nursing practice. *Journal of Advanced Nursing*, **16**, 1090–98.

Johnson, D.E. (1974) Development of theory: a requisite for nursing as a primary health profession. *Nursing Research*, **23**(5), 373–7.

Leddy, S. & Pepper, J. (1989) *Conceptual Bases of Professional Nursing*, 2nd ed. J.B. Lippincott Company, Philadelphia.

Lister, P. (1987) The misunderstood model. *Nursing Times*, **83**(41), 40–42.

Manthey, M. (1980) *The Practice of Primary Nursing*. Blackwell Scientific Publications, Oxford.

May, C. (1992) Nursing work, nurses' knowledge, and the subjectification of the patient. *Sociology of Health & Illness*, **14**(4), 472–87.

Miller, A. (1985) The relationship between nursing theory and nursing practice. *Journal of Advanced Nursing*, **10**(5), 417–24.

Morse, J. (1991) *Qualitative Nursing Research: A Contemporary Dialogue*. Sage Publications, Newbury Park, California.

Orem, D.E. (1991) *Nursing Concepts of Practice*, 4th ed. C.V. Mosby, St Louis.

Pembrey, S. (1984) Nursing care: professional progress. *Journal of Advanced Nursing*, **9**, 539–47.

Pembrey, S. (1989) *Oxford District Health Authority Guidelines for Nursing Practice*. Oxford District Health Authority.

Porter, S. (1991) A participant observation study of power relations between nurses and doctors in a general hospital. *Journal of Advanced Nursing*, **16**, 728–35.

Roper, N., Logan, W.W. & Tierney, A.J. (1980) *The Elements of Nursing*. Churchill Livingstone, Edinburgh.

Roy, C. Sr & Andrews, H.A. (1991) The Roy Adaptation Model: The Definitive

Statement. In: *Conceptual Models for Nursing Practice*, (ed. J.P. Riehl–Sisca). Appleton & Lange, California.

Ryan, D. (1989) *Project 1999 – The Support Hierarchy as the Management Contribution to Project 2000*. Discussion paper, Department of Nursing Studies, University of Edinburgh.

Schon, D.A. (1987) *Educating the Reflective Practitioner: Towards a New Design for Teaching and Learning in the Professions*. Jossey-Bass Publishers, San Francisco.

United Kingdom Central Council for Nursing, Midwifery and Health Visiting (1992) *Code of Professional Conduct*. UKCC, London.

Waterworth, S. & Luker, K. (1990) Reluctant collaborators: do patients want to be involved in decisions concerning care? *Journal of Advanced Nursing*, **15**, 971–76.

Wright, S.G. (1986) *Building and Using a Model of Nursing*. Edward Arnold Publishers, London.

Wright, S.G. (1989) *Changing Nursing Practice*. Edward Arnold Publishers, London.

Editor's commentary

In this chapter Robert Garbett suggests how the cue questions within the BNDU model might be modified to suit the needs of an acute unit. When I developed the model I did not suggest that there was any hierarchy or step-by-step progression within the cue questions, yet clearly the way I have listed the cue questions does reflect some continuity of anticipated events within the patient's care setting career, reflecting the person's anticipated movement through admission towards projected discharge and the continuance of the person's life. The grouping of the cue questions into three areas of assessment begins to offer a more structured approach and shifts the emphasis of the intended cue into a more concrete question requiring a definite answer.

Within this approach, I feel that Robert should include the cue question 'How must this person be feeling?' as a baseline question because it is so central to recognizing the patient as a person. Perhaps this reflects to some extent the different care settings; many patients on 7e are admitted in medical crisis. Failure to include this cue question as a baseline question may symbolically and actually undermine the concept of holism central to the BNDU model.

Robert makes an argument for increasing the range of cue questions by suggesting the extra questions:

'What information does this person need?'
'What additional support might they need?'

The BNDU model cue question 'What support does this person have in life?' subsumes the concept of 'additional' support and focuses the practitioner's attention on the continuity of care outside the immediate care setting. In considering these issues the practitioner will reflect on the level of support *in situ* and additional support that may be desired.

Similarly, paying attention to this cue question will draw the practitioner's attention to actions necessary to ensure an appropriate discharge. Such actions will include the giving of information by paying attention to the cue question 'How can I help this person?' In other words, the cue questions cannot easily be viewed as discrete entities, but are interrelated with each other. They are considered fundamental to all nursing situations.

The breakdown of cue questions into sub-questions, or becoming cue questions in their own right, increases the risk of creating a need for a comprehensive nursing assessment structure that is at once possible of becoming interpreted as a dogmatic and prescriptive assessment strategy as with the assessment strategies in prescriptive models of nursing.

In many respects, such questions and clarification are marginal to using the model in practice. Through reflection and evaluation the model will shape itself to the practice setting. Yet such discussion does reflect the sort of debate that practitioners may need to become involved in to consider the application of the BNDU model.

Chapter 8
Using the BNDU Model in the Community

Susan Metcalf and Christopher Johns

This chapter describes the beginning of a process of evaluating the impact of the BNDU model on my practice as a district nurse. This influence has been profound and has led to a re-assertion of my beliefs and values concerning the nature of district nursing.

The use of models of nursing in my practice

The district nursing team of which I am a member comprises two district nurses, one district enrolled nurse, one newly-qualified staff nurse and three part-time auxiliary nurses. We work in a rural area covering a practice population of approximately 16 000 with a current caseload of approximately 150 patients.

In our practice, as with other teams within the Community NHS Trust, we have used both the Roper, Logan and Tierney (1980) model and the Orem (1980) model. We chose these models because they were the most familiar to us, the easiest to use and most appropriate to our organizational system. For example, Roper *et al.*'s 'activities of living' are reflected in the nature of many of the questions asked on the nursing assessment form which we are required to complete for the FIP nurse management system computer information package.

However, on considering the value of the Roper *et al.* model in the context of my practice, I now perceive it as focusing my attention on seeing the patient as a set of tasks to be done within the discrete activities of living. This is a functional approach to assessment in contrast with the philosophical approach advocated by Johns (1991) which reflects our yet unstated beliefs concerning the nature of our district nursing practice and what this practice aims to achieve. The information gained from filling in some of the boxes is not relevant to nursing many of the patients I work with. My preference has therefore been to use Orem's model as I feel it reflects my perceived complementary role in enabling the patient to undertake self-care.

I find both models can be long-winded and complex and I tend to document only the information which is needed when nursing intervention is required; otherwise much of the information would be irrelevant. However, I feel this is an unsatisfactory practice as it fails to give a good overall picture of the patient. What is required is a concise and relevant assessment and ensuing plan for nursing the patient without having to wade through an excess of information. In other words, pragmatism is an important consideration.

In considering the internal environment of care (Johns 1991), the reality of heavy caseloads emerges as a significant limiting factor to caring for the 'whole person'. If my caseload for the day consists of seeing 25 patients, it is very easy and sometimes very necessary to merely focus on giving the injection, applying the dressing or inserting the catheter. The focus of work can easily become one of controlling the environment in order to get through the work. This leads to defensiveness on the part of the district nurse who knows this is not the desired scenario. So we tend to rationalize our task approach to patients in order to cope, to blame it on the system or even to delude ourselves that we do see and care for the whole patient.

But why do we need to see an overall picture of the patient? As a team we discussed informally our beliefs and values about the nature of nursing in our practice. We have not yet developed our own philosophy for practice and feel that we must explore this further. Indeed, exploring the potential of the BNDU model for our practice has prompted this activity. As Johns (1991) highlights, the use of the BNDU model is dependent on our realization of our collective beliefs and values about district nursing. Johns argues that the sensible use of any model of nursing is based on a compatibility between beliefs and values of practitioners with the assumptions that underpin the model's framework.

I find that using the BNDU model prompts me to constantly reflect on my beliefs and values. As such, these become more and more the basis of my practice rather than a mere orientation to tasks to be accomplished. As an experienced district nurse I ask myself, 'Why do I need to write my beliefs and values down? Isn't it enough to know these "intuitively"? Surely I know what district nursing is.' Johns (1991) argues that writing down answers to these questions makes it more likely that patients receive more consistent and congruent care. From my perspective I agree that we should approach each patient in such a way. This gives direction to new staff and ensures that different nurses who visit a patient approach and respond to the patient in mutually compatible ways.

On reflection, we felt we were in agreement with the BNDU philosophy of care and that it was appropriate and compatible to our practice. In particular, we fundamentally agreed with the concept of a holistic approach that recognizes and values the 'whole person'.

For example, when I apply a dressing, the quality of care is related to my seeing the 'whole person', the person behind the dressing. Anything less than this is to treat the person with disrespect, or in fact not to see them as a person at all but rather as some object I am doing something to. Such is the perversity of task-focused nursing. It is not enough to merely focus on the dressing or delight in my technical mastery of applying it while I subconsciously manipulate the environment to achieve my anticipated exit. I say 'subconsciously' because admitting this fact to myself becomes unacceptable even though I rationalize this action in utilitarian terms of the needs of other patients.

As a consequence of accepting a holistic approach, I become conscious of who I am and of my actions in response to the patient/person with whom I interact. This results in an obvious and conscious shift from a position of manipulating the environment to one of negotiation with the patient. This does not mean that I give control to the patient, but it recognizes the essential worth of 'working with' patients. Obviously environmental factors such as time and pressure to visit other patients, attend meetings, etc. influence this negotiation, but patients know and respect this. It does not require defensive posturing. This shift from manipulation to negotiation is a shift from the dishonesty that underpins any attempts of manipulation.

Anticipatory and adversarial alliances

A negotiated relationship leads to what we call an anticipatory alliance with the patient. We use the word 'anticipatory' because negotiation is based on a mutual knowing of each other's expectations. As such, I and my patients are able to positively anticipate our planned meetings.

I contrast this alliance with an 'adversarial alliance', a term coined by McLaughlin and Carey (1993) in seeking to develop therapeutic relationships between families of brain-injured patients and health care workers. I equate adversarial alliance to manipulation characterized by defensive manoeuvres which hinder caring for patients in a holistic sense. The patient can sense this and though they may say nothing, their body reflects the situation. The result is mutual discomfort which serves to strengthen the adversarial alliance. The visit becomes a suppressed conflict based on uncertainty, mismatched and unarticulated expectations, unmet needs and guardedness. The task is accompanied by compensatory glibness and contradictory words of reassurance and advice as we back towards the door anticipating our controlled exit.

This adversarial relationship is reminiscent of what Robinson and Thorne (1984) refer to as 'guarded alliance' between the nurse and the relative in an attempt to reconstitute a relationship based on minimal conflict where at least some of the relative's needs can be met. The outcome is a blunting of the sensitivity of human caring and a process of mutual diminishment. Both the nurse and the patient are impoverished in the process and both feel less than satisfied by the encounter.

Respecting guests

Obviously the environment of practice at Burford is different from the environment of care in our district nursing practice, with the patient being nursed in their own home rather than in a hospital setting. Away from the depersonalizing environment of the hospital, it is more likely that we are able to see the whole person and it is important that we respect the patient as a person as we are guests in their home. It is equally important to respect patients as people in hospital. The difference is that within the home we are 'invited guests' whereas in hospital the patient is the 'invited guest'. In either case respect must be honoured.

In response to the different care-giving environment, we changed two of the cue questions to reflect this: 'What health event brings this person into hospital?' became 'What health event prompts my visit to this person?', and 'What is important for this person to make their stay in hospital comfortable?' became 'What is important for this person to make my visit comfortable for them?'

Reflections on the use of the BNDU model

On a superficial level we found the BNDU model simple to use and instinctively felt it was a useful tool to assessing the patient. The enrolled nurse and myself thought that the cue questions were actually what we tended to think of when assessing the patient. In this respect, the BNDU model reflected a natural process of our caring rather than asking us to interpret the way we thought about a patient into more complex and alien patterns which the Roper *et al.* and Orem models of nursing were inclined to do. In this way the cue questions helped us to value our natural thoughts and made us both feel more competent and confident in our assessment of patients.

The newly-qualified staff nurse found the cue questions very helpful as she had little experience in assessment. What experience she had had was hospital-focused using models of nursing that she said had little personal meaning to her. From a philosophical perspective this concept of 'personal' meaning is an important consideration in using a model of nursing. I feel that a model has to become an extension of the nurse as a means of relating appropriately with the patient.

By using the BNDU model, our assessments now give a much better overall picture of the patient and clearly lead to recognizing and selecting appropriate interventions to meet the patient's and their family's needs, and for many dependent patients the support to remain in their home.

As a consequence we feel that our care planning has improved as we are now able to pay more attention to the patient's psychological and social needs, and to recognize and understand the impact of our feelings towards the patient in considering how we can help them to meet these needs.

To illustrate the use of the BNDU model in practice I shall use three case studies.

Case study – Patsy: a 'difficult' patient

Patsy was referred to our district nursing team by social services for a 'help bath'. She was known to me as we had visited her to give enemas and dietary advice during episodes of constipation. I had only met Patsy a couple of times as she was a colleague's patient.

She was well known as being a 'difficult' lady and a 'troublemaker'. An article had appeared in the local paper about her not getting enough help as she was housebound. This was felt by us to be very unfair as she was receiving daily homecare. She had also been offered respite care which she cancelled at the last minute. The article gave the impression that she was a very neglected old lady. I felt very negative towards her as I knew of her reputation and the feelings of my colleagues, homecarers and the general practitioner.

When I visited Patsy I found that she was very lonely, she had never married and the only relative she had was a nephew who lived about 40 miles away so she did not see him often. She used to be the local district nurse so she had preconceived ideas about her care. She could not understand that 'times had changed' and she kept saying, 'It was not like this in my day'. She felt that she had got the 'short straw'. She would really have liked to have gone into a residential care home, but she did not see why she should have to use her 'hard earned' savings to contribute to her care.

By using the BNDU model and answering the cue questions, 'How must this person be feeling?' and 'How does this person make me feel?', I gave much more thought to trying to understand Patsy and could talk with her about her feelings and thoughts about the future. It made me conscious of how important it was for me and my colleagues to be aware of our feelings towards this person in order to be able to understand why she was behaving in the way that led us to originally perceive her as 'difficult' and which led me to visit her with preconceived ideas.

Using the cue questions enabled me to explore with Patsy the reasons for her behaviour. As a consequence I could accept this lady for who she was and could understand how she felt about her predicament. Visiting to give her a bath only reinforced her sense of helplessness and loss of control. She needed to be understood and in control of her future.

As a result she responded much more positively towards me, coming to trust me as someone who was genuinely concerned for her rather than as someone to fight against. The experience was a salutary lesson of the perversity of labelling the patient as 'difficult' and how this leads nurses and others to picture a person in such negative terms. I felt very positive to Patsy as a result of my visits to her. What was originally perceived as a threatening and stressful encounter became an enlightening and satis-fying experience.

The profound issue in this experience is:

'Why did it take such simple cue questions to fundamentally reor-ientate myself to practice?'

In trying to make sense of this question I can only draw the conclusion of how blind to caring we can become due to ways of trying to cope with pressures of work. This again reminds me of what Johns (1991) describes as the 'internal environment' – in which nurses and other carers relate to each other in ways that allow the patient to be valued as a person despite the difficulties this sometimes causes.

Recognizing that we do value the whole person makes it essential that we address this issue in our practice. Otherwise we risk leading contradictory lives where our values and our practice are incompatible and we hide behind our rationalizations to protect ourselves.

Case study – Annie

This second case study is focused around introducing the BNDU model to my student district nurse. Her initial reaction was that several visits would have to be made to a patient before an assessment could be completed from which a care plan could be drawn up with the patient. She was not convinced that by using the model we would have enough information to use as a basis for drawing up a care plan with the patient, but she was willing to try it. We visited the patient who was referred to us by the oncology clinic the previous day for dressings to a fungating breast tumour. The student used the cue questions to frame this assessment.

'Who is this person?'

Annie is an 86-year-old lady who has been widowed for a 'few' years. She has one daughter and two grandchildren. Her only sister died about six months previously of a breast carcinoma. She has recently moved into a 'granny annexe' in her daughter's home. She says she doesn't really miss where she used to live as she hadn't many friends there anyway.

'What health event has prompted my visit to this person?'

She was referred to us from the oncology clinic to assess her needs and redress a fungating breast carcinoma. Annie told us that she first noticed a discharge from her breast about six years ago but she hoped it would go away, and anyway she was far too busy looking after her husband and then her sister to bother with it. Once she had moved into her new flat her daughter noticed it and immediately took her to the general practitioner. He immediately referred her on to the oncology clinic, but did not refer her to us as the daughter said she was quite happy to redress the wound herself. The oncology clinic were not happy with the dressings and felt that Annie would benefit from having visits from us.

'How must this person be feeling?'

She appears to be fairly cheerful and says she doesn't want to be a bother.

'How had this event affected her usual life patterns and roles?'

It doesn't appear to be affecting her life pattern at present, apart from requiring regular visits from us. She says she likes being at home and at the moment doesn't want to go out and socialize. In her previous home she said that neither she nor her husband went out very much.

'How does this person make me feel?'

On first impression she is a very pleasant, likeable old lady. I feel sad that she was not referred to us earlier as we could have made her feel much more comfortable with a more appropriate dressing.

'How can I help this person?'

By redressing her breast as appropriate to make her feel comfortable. I can also refer her to other agencies as required and give support to her and her family.

'What is important for this person to make my visit comfortable for her?'

This is difficult to answer after only one visit. Annie said she would be pleased to see us any day at any time – whatever suited us best.

'What support does this person have?'

Annie lives in close proximity to her daughter and family. It means that there are family around her when she needs them, but she can also continue to lead an independent life. She is alone all day as her daughter works. She is able to do her household chores with the help of a weekly private cleaner. She cooks for herself but joins the family for Sunday lunch. Her daughter shops for her but Annie is able to walk to the local shop. We shall be visiting daily at present to redress her breast.

'How does she view the future for herself and others?'

On first impression Annie does not seem to be looking a long way into the future. She is waiting to go into hospital for a mastectomy which she is dreading. She says she will be 'glad when it is all over and she is back home'.

From this initial assessment which only took 45 minutes we were able to draw up a care plan which on the next visit we showed Annie and asked if she agreed or wanted to add anything. The student was surprised at the detail we were able to give when answering the questions after only one visit and how simple the model was to use.

Some questions were difficult to answer, for example, 'How must this person be feeling?', 'How does this person make me feel?', and, 'What is important for this person to make my visit comfortable for her?' We both felt we needed to know Annie and her family better to be able to answer these questions. However, we both felt happy that we could build on this initial assessment on subsequent visits.

The student's difficulty with the cue questions concerning feelings reinforces the comments I made in the first case study. Yet we both felt more satisfied with our work having recognized our own and the patient's feelings. Without doubt this recognition was essential in developing a relationship with Annie.

I find it difficult to write negative feelings about a patient and find it hard to tell a patient I don't like them, especially if I have no particular reason. I believe that a patient should be shown what has been written about them, and in one respect this is inevitable because the notes are left with the patient. Of course the questions are only cue questions and do not need 'concrete' answers. They are only there to simultaneously tune the nurse into their beliefs about nursing and the patient.

This highlights a potential initial difficulty of using the model with the way I have been socialized into using models in a passive and deterministic way. Boxes are meant to be filled in! The reality of the BNDU model is that the nurse needs to be intelligent in using it in the sense that the model is merely a tool towards helping to nurse patients more effectively rather than a task in itself which needs completing. Therefore, the nurse should not write whether they like or dislike the patient, but rather *why* they feel that way.

For example, in the first case study I could write in the patient's care plan:

'Patsy feels lonely and anxious about the cost of moving into residential care. Our aim is to understand how she feels about her present situation and the future and to help her make the best decision.'

In this way I reflect my feelings into a positive channel. I also help my colleagues to deal with their negative feelings towards Patsy. I think that several visits should be made to the patients to establish a relationship in order for them to tell the nurse about themselves and especially how they feel about their situation.

Although we did not challenge Annie's perceptions of her health situation on the first visit, the information gained from her highlighted many potential issues about her future that we needed to bear in mind in our visits. It was also interesting to note how she quickly adapted to her envisaged patient role by saying we could visit at any time that 'suited us'. We could always check with her that our visiting times were mutually convenient.

Case study – Connie

The third case study is an account of my first use of the BNDU model to reassess a patient I had been nursing for four years. Although I realized the cue questions were designed to enable me to approach the patient in a way compatible with my beliefs and values, I used the questions to structure the assessment. I felt this was necessary as the BNDU approach seemed alien in comparison with my previous experience of the Roper *et al.* and Orem models.

'Who is this person?'

Connie is 74 years old and lives alone in a council-owned bungalow. She has three living children. One son died in a road accident many years ago. One daughter lives in Australia and she writes regularly. The other daughter lives locally and gives her a lot of help. Her son also lives locally, but he does not visit his mother often.

'What health event has prompted my visit to this person?'

Over the last four years Connie has had many admissions to hospital for treatment for arterial sclerosis. She has had both legs amputated above the thigh. Now she is wheelchair-bound.

'How must this person be feeling?'

Connie says that she feels 'useless' and hates having to rely on others to help her with personal and household tasks. She does get tearful at times and gets anxious if she is unwell as she does not want to be admitted to hospital again. Her husband left home six months ago following a family argument. She is very upset as they have been married for 54 years. However, she has since confided that the marriage had not been a happy one. She says that in a way she is relieved that he has left, although 'it is still upsetting after all those years together'. Now she is worried in case he walks in, as she insists she does not want him back. She is having to get used to living alone, but she says that it has not been too difficult as he was out for much of the day and evening. She doesn't feel lonely as her neighbours, friends and daughter are visiting her more often now.

'How has this event affected her life patterns and roles?'

Over the years Connie has adapted to being in a wheelchair. She now has a microwave oven which has enabled her to cook, as she was finding it too difficult using a conventional oven. This has helped a lot as her husband used to lift saucepans off and on the cooker for her. She can also manage simple household tasks such as dusting and ironing which she does enjoy doing and says she has always been very house-proud.

Her home has been adapted to meet some of her needs, for example, a raised toilet seat and frame and a monkey pole and bedlocks that help her to get in and out of bed more easily. She is now unable to go out without help but she says she is happy to stay at home. She says she cannot get into a car now so her outings are restricted to going for walks locally and to her daughter's home. She has only recently been able to do this as she has a urinary catheter *in situ*. At first when she had the catheter she wasn't very keen but now she is delighted as it has given her the freedom to go out, whereas before she could only use the toilet at her home.

Connie thoroughly enjoys knitting and crocheting and is thankful she is still able to do this.

'How can I help this person?'

I can help Connie by listening to her problems and advising her. I visit weekly to help her wash and dress, to check that her pressure areas are intact and give catheter care.

'What is important for this person to make my visit comfortable for them?'

Connie likes to know which member of the team is visiting. She likes her visits to be as near to 9 o'clock [in the morning] as possible as she does not like being in her nightclothes in her wheelchair. She realizes that this might not be possible every visit as we may have to see other patients early. We always let her know approximately what time we will visit and she always appreciates this.

'What support does this person have?'

Connie receives a lot of help from the district nurses, social services, family and friends. She is visited daily by either the district nursing team or home-carers. We alternate to help Connie wash and dress daily. Home-care also gives her an hour a week to clean the bungalow and change her bedding. Her friends and neighbour help her with the washing and any other jobs that home-care may not have had time to do, such as cleaning the windows.

Her daughter does all her shopping and also prepares some meals for her. Connie goes every Sunday to her daughter's home. She always contacts her daily by phone or personally to make sure that she is comfortable and has had everything she needs. Connie is always appreciative of this care as the daughter also works and she says that she has her own life to lead.

'How does she view the future for herself and others?'

Connie is concerned about the future. She says that she wonders what will happen to her when she can no longer transfer from her wheelchair. She wants to stay in her own home, but if ever the time comes when she cannot look after herself she does not want to go into residential care. She has discussed this with her daughters and they have both told her they would look after her in their own homes. She is relieved about this, but she says she doesn't want to be a burden to them.

Over a period of time it is easy to take for granted aspects of patients' care and to become complacent about one's helping role. This example illustrates the ease with which I used the BNDU model. The cue questions helped me review Connie's total care and putting it all down on paper also made the information available to my colleagues, enabling them to see Connie as I saw her. However, it may take myself and my colleagues some time to adjust to writing in this 'narrative' style.

It is interesting to reflect on the question, 'How has this event affected her life patterns and roles?' Thinking about Roper *et al.*'s activities of living, I would look at the issues surrounding mobility, eating, sleeping, eliminating, working and playing that complement each other. Initially I did wonder whether the structure of the BNDU model would give a detailed-enough assessment. Clearly my fears were unfounded. Rather than these issues being discrete activities they now merged into a wholeness that made immediate sense. The focus on wholeness was maintained and yet the detail remained intact.

Neither the Roper *et al.* model nor the Orem model really encouraged us to reflect on who the person was in this holistic sense. Neither did they encourage a focus on psychological or social aspects of caring. The emphasis on universal self-care requisites and activities of living is physically orientated. Also, the wording of Orem's more psycho–social self-care requisites is obscure and difficult to interpret.

Organizational consequences of using the BNDU model

Using the model has prompted a review of the amount and relevance of the material demanded by the FIP computer system. In this sense the BNDU model is empowering because its reflective nature encourages the team to challenge and take control of practice in a positive rather than in a reactive or defensive way.

The model has certainly helped us to reflect on our beliefs and values regarding the essential nature of district nursing practice. This is an important issue not just in the sense of giving care to patients. It relates back to what Johns (1991) refers to as the 'external environment' and questioning the purpose of district nursing. Writing this chapter has helped me to put some of these issues into personal perspective.

The external environment of practice is radically changing in organizational terms with the advent of general practitioner fundholding and trusts. In this climate, district nurses must be able to assert the nature of their role.

With the implementation of the Community Care Act 1993 there have been changes affecting the way in which we give care in the community. A pilot project was undertaken to look into care management and one of the conclusions was the need for a good assessment of the patient by an assessor who was not connected with health or social services. There was also a need for shared documentation to prevent duplication of information. I discussed the potential of the BNDU model with the pilot project coordinator for use as the basis for assessment. We both felt that we needed to pursue the possibility as it seemed to us an ideal model which could have multi-disciplinary uses.

Conclusions

As a team I realize that we need a philosophy of nursing. We have discussed the BNDU philosophy and we agree with it, but it does need some adapting for our environment of practice. I hope that our district nursing group will do this and, as a result, more nurses will use the BNDU model.

At present we keep the completed assessments rather than leaving them with the patients in their homes. This is very helpful, particularly when visiting a patient for the first time as an associate nurse; the assessments give a good overall picture of the patient. They have been written concisely and are easy to read, giving the relevant information to be able to nurse the patient effectively.

Inevitably the work described in this chapter only gives partial attention to the development of the BNDU model in our district nursing practice. It is difficult to explain how such a seemingly simple model can renurture such a sense of commitment in me towards nursing; it has enabled and empowered me to at once voice, value and enact my caring beliefs. And it is not just me. The model is viewed with considerable hope and optimism by my colleagues as a framework for guiding practice. Over time, environmental factors have a limiting effect on caring potential. The model helps to re-focus the meaning of district nursing and in the process nurtures caring beliefs.

The ideas in this chapter are a reflection of my dialogue with Christopher Johns helping me to make sense of the model. He felt it was important that I make this contribution to the book because so often such books are written by theorists rather than by ordinary practitioners reflecting on their struggle to make sense of their practice and emergent theory. I have never been critical before of either my practice or theory. Though aware of the coming and going of other theories, I have taken refuge in my habitualized practice.

I make this point in order to give courage to other practitioners who feel oppressed by or who shelter from reflection on their practice. We all have a responsibility to develop our practice in order to meet the needs of our patients more effectively. This of course assumes that nurses do want to care for their patients. Without doubt, to embrace the BNDU model is to embrace human caring as the core of nursing. Yet, as I hope I have illustrated, that embrace opens the door to mutual ways of working with patients and mutual satisfaction within our caring relationships. In this way, we are all winners.

References

Johns, C.C. (1991) The Burford Nursing Development Unit holistic model of nursing practice. *Journal of Advanced Nursing*, **16**, 1090–98.

McLaughlin, A.M. & Carey, J.L. (1993) The adversarial alliance: developing therapeutic relationships between families and the team in brain injury rehabilitation. *Brain Injury*, **7**(1), 45–59.

Orem, D.E. (1980) *Nursing Concepts of Practice*. McGraw-Hill Book Company, New York.

Robinson, C.A. & Thorne, S.E. (1984) Strengthening patient interference. *Journal of Advanced Nursing*, **9**, 597–602.

Roper, N., Logan, W.W. & Tierney, A.J. (1980) *The Elements of Nursing*. Churchill Livingstone, Edinburgh.

Editor's commentary

This chapter has illustrated how written assessments can be expressed using the cue questions as if they are questions requiring definite answers. Without doubt, practitioners will use the cue questions in this 'concrete' way until they have been internalized and become part of how the practitioners 'naturally' view their practice.

It remains to be seen whether Susan Metcalf is able to influence the current nursing input into the FIP system. Her experience highlights how such systems reduce practitioners to slaves, i.e. inputting useless information without any benefit, as if to say, 'We have invested in this technology and you will use it regardless'.

In busy work lives, practitioners need tools that are useful in their day-to-day practice. The cue questions direct or tune the practitioner into the key aspects of their practice and, as such, whilst reflective and challenging, they are also pragmatic.

Chapter 9
Julia Farr Centre Nursing Development Unit: A Model for Practice

Bart O'Brien and Judith Pope

In 1991 the Nursing Department of Julia Farr Centre (JFC), a 500-bed extended care setting in Adelaide, South Australia, endorsed the establishment of a Nursing Development Unit (NDU). The work of the Centre had been influenced by the report of the Future Directions Working Party (Glass 1989). This recommended, amongst other things, that long-term care admissions and the general-purpose nursing home focus of the Centre be changed to create a range of living options for a predominantly younger, disabled population with care requirements mainly stemming from the effects of Acquired Brain Damage, often traumatically acquired.

A changing focus of care at Julia Farr Centre has been a precipitating factor in the evolution of the NDU. Other external factors impacting on the NDU include social demand for increasingly effective and efficient responses to the range of complex nursing needs associated with caring for people affected by a variety of neurological conditions.

In 1993 the NDU's population included people with medical diagnoses of multiple sclerosis, rheumatoid arthritis, brain stem CVA and traumatic brain damage. (See Fig. 9.1 – the nursing needs admission profile, developed in late 1991). The NDU is an on-campus ward with 20 commissioned beds whose occupancy levels are regulated by the dependency levels of people admitted. Dependency is determined by the Centre's Nursing Information System (Spry & O'Brien 1993) and reflects the person's requirements for nursing care.

The conceptual framework that initially evolved from the reflective interpretation of NDU nurses' experience at Julia Farr Centre has come to be challenged through an evolving dialogue, established between Christopher Johns and the authors of this chapter. The commitment to reflective practice has encouraged nurses to interpret and articulate their own evolving practice rather than slavishly adopting the dictates of a particular nursing model.

(1)   Residents who have suffered cerebral trauma and have sub-acute nursing needs, e.g.

    1.1   Tracheostomy tube *in situ* – with potential for extubation.
    1.2   Gastrostomy tube *in situ* – with potential for transitional feeding program.
    1.3   Altered swallowing ability – with potential for improvement.
    1.4   Unstable physical condition, i.e. blood pressure, skin actions, diabetic state – with potential to stabilize.
    1.5   Serial plastering of limbs – with potential for correct limb alignment.

(2)   The resident's return to the community is considered a physical, emotional and social improbability in the short-term (9–12 months).
(3)   The resident has a supportive family/significant other(s) who is/are interested in restorative care and who will become an integral part of the group effort to provide such care.
(4)   The resident requires predominantly nursing care with a degree of medical consultation.
(5)   Allied health input will be on a consultative basis until the resident reaches the stage where intensive, consistent allied health input is required to maximize self-fulfilment and independence. Physiotherapy, speech therapy, occupational therapy plus recreational therapy, social work input and services of the Centre chaplain are the predominant allied health contributions.
(6)   Residents who have the potential to improve mentally and physically will progress primarily to other wards/services for further stimulation or to other suitable alternative accommodation or to the community.
(7)   With some residents it may become apparent that they would no longer benefit from the NDU program. In such cases, after being brought to the highest achievable level of function, arrangements will be made for transfer to alternative lifestyle accommodation (extended care).
(8)   Discharge from the NDU will be on the basis of the achievement of resident and nursing objectives, resident individual progress, the feelings of the resident and family or significant other(s), discussion with the NDU Senior Clinician (Clinical Nurse Consultant – CNC), and other appropriate accommodation/community representative(s).
(9)   Residents meeting the Admission Profile will be referred to the NDU by the Centre's Assessment Ward or Admission Panel, by interested relatives/significant other(s), Parent Support Group, or by CNCs of other wards/care areas. The NDU CNC will undertake a nursing assessment, against this criteria, prior to discussion with the Unit team (Assistant Director of Nursing, Clinical, Medical Officer, ward Clinical Nurses, ward allied health consultants) and the NDU Family Support Group.

Fig. 9.1   The NDU admission profile.

Arising out of this discourse came the decision:

'... to construct a tailor-made model of nursing from the practitioner's own values and beliefs...' (Johns 1991, p.1091).

The focus of this chapter then, is the initial reflection on considering the value of the BNDU model for nursing practice within the practice setting of the Julia Farr Centre Nursing Development Unit.

Nursing models are stylized imitations of nursing practice. A model is a way of looking at and organizing things to make them meaningful:

'It "simplifies" reality, narrowing one's attention to specific concerns.... By its very nature, a model reflects the culture and milieu of the times and incorporates implicit values. Thus, to understand, analyse and evaluate a given model it is necessary to identify its philosophical underpinnings.' (Feild & Winslow 1985)

A significant factor in developing clinical practice at the Julia Farr Centre NDU was to define and articulate practice in the Unit. Earlier research into developing and evolving nursing practice (B.B. O'Brien, unpublished observations) suggested that the foundations for a conceptual framework lay in articulation of a philosophy for nursing. In this exercise the NDU undertook to identify and interpret two forms of understanding that Brand (1984) calls declarative and procedural knowledge.

Declarative knowledge is the understanding that provides the ability to readily answer questions such as, 'What do you call that?' The answer is recalled from memory, perhaps in reference to some association framework. However, the answer to the question, 'How do you do that?', is much harder to articulate and is the result of procedural knowledge. Generally it is much easier to demonstrate the answer to this sort of question than it is to verbally describe the steps and principles involved.

Brand describes the process of acquiring both sets of knowledge as one where ability to 'perform' an activity was initially learned at a declarative level. As the taught steps become internalized with practice they may have become subject to changes fashioned by context and resources. The consequence in outcome is that there can frequently be important differences and simplifications between what is said and what is done, or, in other words, a potential for a theory–practice gap, particularly as changing practice in the Unit led staff to adapt and redesign skills learnt in very different settings.

In exploring the issues that arose from trying to find and eliminate the tensions or differences arising when Unit procedural knowledge does not match the Unit's declared intent, the decision was taken to use critical theory to guide and structure the Unit's evolving conceptual framework.

Critical theory (Fay 1975) challenges practitioners to make sense of all observed behaviour because all actions, which manifest as observed behaviour, are taken towards achieving specific outcomes and are implicitly meaningful for practitioners and clients and as such cannot be taken for granted. Critical theory also recognizes that the actions of practitioners are influenced by their social environment over which they may feel they have either little understanding or feel powerless to change. Also, many actions by practitioners and clients are unanticipated; they arise as a result of an unconscious reaction to the environment.

Fay emphasizes how the interconnection of practice and theory is such that what is recognized as being 'fact' (truth) is determined through reflection on actions, in contrast with the traditional science view where 'fact' is prescribed and directs action, and as a consequence tends to be non-reflective.

The recognition of the value of critical theory as a philosophical paradigm to guide the development of a conceptual framework for NDU practice has served to focus attention on NDU beliefs and behaviours and has enabled NDU nurses to scrutinize proposed theoretical ideas, such as the BNDU model, before they are accepted into NDU thinking.

The need to determine relevance of theory to practice settings has not been lost on nurse practitioners. Greenwood (1984, p.77) states that:

'Clinical nurses do not perceive research findings as relevant to their practice ... because frequently they are not relevant to their practice.'

Happily, even as she was writing these words, a body of clinically-based research was being undertaken in the UK, intended to better integrate theory and practice to develop new norms in nursing practice. Alan Pearson's developmental work (1983; 1988) with nursing units at Burford, Oxford and Geelong (Australia), together with the work of other nurses associated with such units, (Wright 1989; J. Salvage, unpublished observations; Johns 1991; B.B. O'Brien, unpublished observations) suggests that working outside nursing's traditional epistemological association with its allegiance to medical and empirical science can extend and expand nurses' understanding of their potential therapeutic contribution.

The BNDU model – application in the JFC NDU

The remainder of this contribution is an attempt to filter an evolving understanding of nursing practice through the components of the BNDU model. In doing so, there is recognition of the debt that both Units owe to Pearson's seminal work in this field, as well as to the contributions of the many nurses who have further developed his original belief in the therapeutic contribution that can attend a restructuring of nursing practice.

The BNDU model (Johns 1991) conceptual framework has served to organize a number of concepts central to nursing in the JFC NDU (Fig. 9.2). An initial conceptual framework included elements from a number

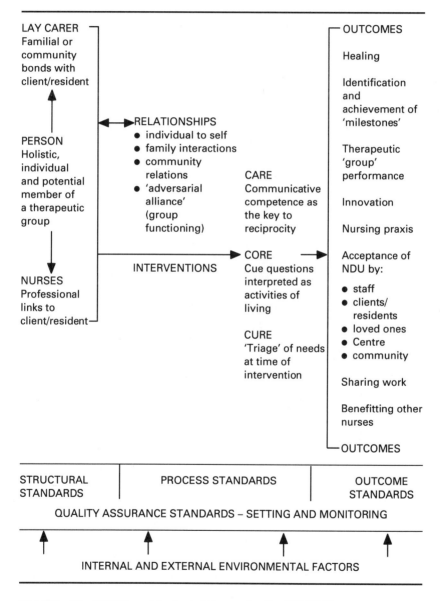

Fig. 9.2 The BNDU model adapted for use by the JFC NDU.

of nursing models and served to introduce to NDU nurses how conceptualizing and articulating their practice could aid in further understanding of its potential. Reformulation of the major elements of that framework, using the BNDU model, served to illustrate how different conceptualizations lend different emphasis to various elements. This was an important discovery and has led to serious reflection on the practical, as opposed to espoused, value of the elements of the initial framework. The model illustrated above suggests current JFC NDU thinking and the remainder of this chapter is devoted to explaining Unit practice through the adapted BNDU model.

Philosophy of caring

Nursing practice is grounded in a philosophical statement that in itself rests in a belief system which recognizes the worth and contributions of individuals equally, be they lay or professional carers or the focus of such care. A collaborative approach to care is promoted in which professional carers, lay carers and residents are empowered to contribute equally according to the potential of each group.

Caring in the Unit is orientated to the particular issues and constraints that face people on admission and this has led to the Unit defining health in terms of people's ability to come to terms with their changed circumstances and regain control of their lives. The responsibility of NDU caring activities is focused by this definition of health and includes lay and professional carers and residents as co-participants in the development and implementation of therapies.

Recognition is given to the rights of residents to a lifestyle and environment that promotes interaction with the general community to the fullest extent possible. The staff of the NDU assert that care is focused on the individual and lifestyle and restorative forms of care are offered that reflect the resident's state of independence.

Residents are encouraged to strive for strengthening in areas of weakness and to develop areas of strength, thus enabling them to regain and maintain independence in a safe, caring, homelike environment.

Facilitators of practice

Care standards

Care standards are readily identifiable at Unit, Centre and professional levels. There is a clear commitment by lay and professional carers to the principles of quality assurance, and the use of critical reflection as a catalyst for praxis is central to this commitment.

Organization

Methods of organizing nursing focus on the primary team concept have been adapted to function most effectively within the constraints of the human resources available to the Unit. The involvement of lay carers and other professionals enhances the nursing focus on each person and the impact on their activities of living of the injury or disease process affecting them. The primary nursing team developed in recognition of the issues of commitment and stress associated with primary allocation in extended care where a primary nurse would work with a group of individuals exclusively, possibly for years at a time.

There are two primary teams at any one time, comprised of a team leader and a number of team members plus a small number of 'float staff' who are rostered to keep the two teams functional across the two day shifts, seven days a week, (there is a separate night duty roster). Each primary team has a specific resident population as its primary care focus for a period of two months, after which members are reallocated to opposite teams or to the 'float' pool.

Experience over the past two years suggests that two months is sufficient to promote consistency and commitment to care development without staff burn-out related to the slow rate of change and intensity of nursing NDU residents. Decisions about nursing care are made within each primary team with inter-team communication a feature of the shift to shift handover period. The team leaders (primary nurses) are clinical nurses (Registered General Nurses (RGN), three-year program, with advanced skills and knowledge in NDU nursing) while team members (associate nurses) are either Registered General Nurses or Enrolled General Nurses (one-year program). The option of primary nursing with all RGN staff has been canvassed several times since the NDU's inception, but the Centre does not have resources to provide all RGN staff to a single ward.

Multi-disciplinary team

As with many rehabilitation programs, the NDU has a multi-disciplinary team which meets to discuss and review the contributions and commitment of professional carers to the NDU. As described by Pearson (1988), access to such a team is important if the extensive range of care options such a group can provide are to be regularly canvassed. The NDU multi-disciplinary team responds and monitors nursing requests for consultancy.

Reflective practice

Reflective practice is critical to the transformation of nursing practice into praxis (informed action intended to better the therapeutic potential of caring activities). Issues of nurse management of stress and the effect of stress levels on reflective potential are important to the type of nursing experience common in the NDU, where developing an 'adversarial alliance' (McLaughlin & Carey 1993) is often a precursor to group performance. The importance of communicative competence and communication forums is grounded on the use of critical reflection as a means of understanding why people behave and respond as they do, and as a means of making sense of the outcomes of interpersonal interactions.

As Schon (1983) explains, reflection-in-action can be a powerful learning experience as the person reflecting comes to better understand the effects and implications of their actions. Reflection-on-action, a process somewhat akin to nursing process, is a broader, retrospective analysis of expected and unexpected outcomes of NDU practice. Considered in these two ways, concurrent and retrospective reflective practice has the potential to identify and correct anomalies between nurses' beliefs about nursing and their actual practice.

Compatible models

Elements from compatible models of nursing have been identified by NDU nurses as helping to conceptualize and articulate their own experiential knowledge. There is no slavish allegiance to an external nursing model and the conceptual framework of the NDU model is grounded in the experiences and understanding of Unit nurses. Having said this, there is a clear acknowledgement of the common philosophical grounding of the Burford and JFC NDUs and an awareness that the BNDU model of care, like the JFC NDU conceptual framework, is grounded in the reflective understanding of nurse clinicians.

Clinical leadership

Clinical leadership has been vital to development of the JFC NDU. Alison Kitson's PhD thesis (A.L. Kitson, unpublished observations) has been a seminal reference for its identification of the pivotal role played by the senior clinician in promoting nursing's therapeutic potential.

People – lay and professional carers

For NDU nurses, a basic assumption is that people are people first and nurses or residents, husbands, friends or daughters second. A central feature of NDU practice that has been derived from this is an understanding that care activities stem from and are aimed at members of a special 'group' which forms as the result of a change in health to the person who forms the main focus of that group. Acknowledgement of the need for such a group represents both a challenge to and support for potential group members.

Prior to the obvious need for a care group, it is assumed that the central person had an existence where control of many activities of living was not only self directed but private. There is a further assumption that the person's family interacted in a special way just as, finally, the person and their family maintained a working association with the community where they lived. Note that this model assumes a series of levels of awareness about the activities of the core individual, the relationship of that person with family and the relationships of that family with their immediate community.

The advent of severe brain damage or the onset of a degenerative neurological condition is considered by the NDU to create a severe challenge to the intra- and interpersonal relationships of the normative social group. Suddenly strangers and family are given or assume to make *carte blanche* decisions about body function or maintenance that were previously personally or familiarly private. Nurses, often total strangers, begin to participate in activities of hygiene and toileting; they are present and often contribute to or intervene as advocates in what used to be intra-family business.

For NDU nurses, realization of the implications of such a breakdown in normative social relationships, in the context of the sort of changes to health that precipitated such action, has been the subject of considerable debate. Articulation of the NDU's problem and a working solution has been aided by the work of Kitson (1987). She described the comparative qualities and morality of caring as experienced by professional and lay carers in terms that helped make sense of the confusion and anger that was disabling the team approach to care that had been the NDU's traditional pattern of practice. Since early 1992 the NDU has espoused and worked towards the effective functioning of a group rather than a team approach to nursing care. This group approach focuses caring into lay and professional caring domains with secondary emphasis placed on whether the carer is a nurse or a family member, resident or medical officer.

Kitson (1987) identifies three characteristics of professional care – commitment, possession of a body of knowledge and skills, and professional integrity – that are considered basic to the role of the professional carer. Lay carers' empowerment, in their extensive knowledge of the person's personal and social functioning, is frequently much more implicit and subservient, often overshadowed by assumptions about the functioning of health services coupled with often conflicting demands on the resources of lay carers by work and their continuing social commitments. The commitment of NDU nurses is to provide lay carers with opportunities to add their intensely personalized care to the professional contribution. Combined with their background knowledge, lay carers are ideally placed to reflect on developments in and the effects of care activities. In an acute but long-term rehabilitation setting these contributions are an extremely valuable contribution to the NDU's skill and knowledge base.

Relationships

Relationships between people associated with the NDU are grounded on a holistic understanding of people as individuals who are potential members of a therapeutic group.

Use of the term 'group' is a deliberate attempt to move away from language that tends to disempower lay carers. NDU nurses believe that the concept of team nursing or team caring carries with it an implication that a team of professionals is involved. There may also be an assumption that one team makes decisions for a group of clients or patients. The espoused role of each NDU 'group' is to identify and draw together the relevant, available caring resources required to make the need for the group redundant as quickly as possible. The challenge for each group is to establish a therapeutic relationship between group members that minimizes the potential for adversarial beliefs to jeopardize group reflection on its reason for existence.

Group processes

A group's formation begins as a function of the pre-admission assessment, and consultation with all potential carers is central to this process. Nurses refer to group formation as a procession through the stages of forming, storming, norming, performing and mourning.

Forming occurs as part of the process of assessment and admission to the NDU. At this point the expectations of future group members are coloured by recent experiences of the health system or by interactions with people representing other groups, teams or disciplines. NDU experience is that the forming stage represents a 'honeymoon' period when politeness and courtesy are demonstrated in fairly formal exchanges between members as the group's boundaries and membership become defined.

Storming regularly emerges as the next stage of group development and reflects the identification of a need for an 'adversarial alliance'. In this stage, group members struggle to reconcile the circumstances in which they find themselves with their perceived, expected and unexpected contributions to group performance. There are special needs for lay and professional carers in this stage. For example, as McLaughlin and Carey (1993, p.46) describe:

'Clinicians often hear family comments which address the following:

"If you would give him more therapy, he would get better."
"I resent your nurturing role – I feel helpless."
"I am devastated by my loss – to which you have become a party."
"You are giving up on him."'

Group formation represents a challenge to empower all potential members of the group so that they and other group members acknowledge each person's particular contributions in terms of commitment, knowledge, skills and resources.

Professionals are empowered through social assumptions of their role in managing health care, but are disempowered in relation to their limited knowledge of the particular needs of each individual. While all professional carers, nursing especially, have access to human and material resources often denied to lay carers, the use of these resources is rarely available on a one-to-one basis. Added stressors for professional carers in the storming stage relate to their ability to absorb and accurately reflect these lay carer challenges as the group starts to form.

In the *norming* and *performing* stages of group performance the adversarial alliance reaches its therapeutic potential. Group members have increasing awareness of each other's potential areas of contribution and set standards against which they measure the performance of other members. The performing stage is rarely totally free from the effects of stress, grief and anger, but increasingly the group develops strategies to help individuals as they experience these symptoms.

The *mourning* stage begins when the group begins to realize that the NDU's resources for care provision are being outgrown. Mourning may be manifested in family or significant others' verbalized concerns about being moved out of the Unit or they may show up in nurses' demonstration of caring behaviours that become increasingly accepting of group 'storms', once a discharge or transfer date has been agreed. For lay carers, mourning seems to involve a process of becoming more attached to the NDU, perhaps along the reasoned lines of 'Better the devil you know...'

There is frequent acknowledgement of the benefits that group functioning has brought, coupled with intense questioning about what the future will hold. Often for the first time, any adversarial component to group relationships is lost to a need to prepare for what comes next. For nurses, mourning may bring a sense of wistfulness as they begin to recognize that, ahead of the dissolution of this group, lies the forming and storming process of another, with all the stressors implied in the repetitive cycle of professional care provision.

Sub groups in the NDU

While the group concept is central to the NDU's philosophy of an empowering, cooperative approach to caring practices, it should be recognized that members of each group have work and support networks that cross group boundaries.

Family Carers Group

This group was facilitated by the NDU Clinical Nurse Consultant, initially to provide a forum for information sharing, discussion of issues of concern, support and comfort for the supporters. An initial meeting discussed the grief process, common issues, general information sharing and problem solving as a group. The philosophy of the NDU was also shared. Subsequent meetings have discussed the process of establishing the NDU to ensure that carers are kept informed and have opportunities to comment and give feedback on the effects of introduced change. A carers' information folder was established and many carers and staff contribute their ideas and beliefs through this feedback mechanism. The NDU also has a Unit Journal where comments and records of progress are documented.

The initial meetings of the Family Carers Group proved so successful that it was agreed to schedule subsequent meetings on a three-monthly basis. The NDU Clinical Nurse Consultant acts as recorder and facilitator to enable the members of this group to identify and work through issues and ideas. However, this group is very independent and provides support and a voice for new and veteran lay carers.

Work by Johns (1993) sheds new light on some of the issues associated with integrating these stresses within relationships with the challenge of producing therapeutic outcomes. Johns identifies four domains of learning for the effective primary nurse, which arguably apply to any carer. The first three domains – becoming patient-centred, working therapeutically with patients and giving and receiving feedback – should be familiar to most readers. Johns' fourth domain – coping with work – opens up the carer's responsibilities to include accountability for: recognizing and accepting stress; getting support; and developing therapeutic relationships within the nursing team (NDU group).

The existence of a dialectic between stress levels and reflective competence suggested by Newell (1993) is worth considering here in the face of nursing's increasing commitment to the use of reflection as a part of nursing process. For NDU nurses, the importance of stress management is seen not only in the light of the effect on individual quality of life, but also from a therapeutic perspective where managing stress levels ensures that reflection and reason can continue to be built into patterns of caring practice. One key outcome has been establishing effective communication between the separate lay and professional discourses.

Lay and professional discourses

Research involving the NDU (B.B. O'Brien, unpublished observations) suggests the existence of two significant clinical discourses within the Centre's practice: a lay discourse and a professional discourse. These two discourses, although separately informed by the experience base and belief systems of lay and professional carers respectively, also share common understandings. The need for effective communication between these discourses is crucial to care within the Centre.

The model of lay and professional discourses acknowledges the opportunities for informal as well as formal communication forums where lay–to–lay, lay–to–professional and professional–to–professional contacts occur. Research validated by co-participants suggests that informal contacts, colloquially referred to as 'corridor communications', occur at two levels or for two reasons. A need to release pent-up emotions or concerns immediately can lead individuals to seek out a member of staff. A measure of the continuing effectiveness of NDU functioning can be determined through assessment of the extent to which the formal communication forums act as venues for cathartic expression of concerns, and as venues for problem solving and action planning.

When elements of either activity are seen to be occurring in any of a variety of the informal opportunities for communication that occur from day to day, then an urgent review of the disparities between lay and professional discourses is called for. For the NDU itself and for the development and effective functioning of the group concept, communicative competence is a skill that requires constant attention.

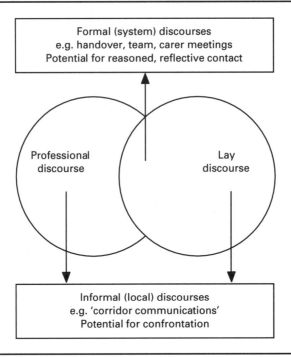

Fig. 9.3   Outcomes of lay and professional discourses in the NDU.

Communicative competence

A key issue within the BNDU adapted framework is the concept of communicative competence towards establishing open and reciprocal relationships between all carers.

NDU research (O'Brien 1992) suggests that reflective practitioners have the task of attempting to reconcile the role of nurse-as-carer with that of nurse-as-person. A potential exists for problems to occur when the belief systems of one role are accorded status based on the authority of the other. For example, a personal belief about a dressing technique might be considered as authoritative based on an understanding that the person espousing the technique is a senior clinician rather than on reflection of whether the principles of the proposed technique hold up under scrutiny. Lack of differentiation between personal and professional (or lay) caring beliefs is conceptualized in the NDU through Habermas' (1987) identification of, and distinction between, the 'lifeworld' of the person and the 'system' in which they function.

We are rarely critical of the vast amount of information we process as we make seemingly simple decisions from day to day. It is, as Habermas reminds us:

'... so unproblematic that we are simply incapable of making ourselves conscious of this or that part of it at will.' (Pusey 1987, p.58)

The task of critical self-reflection is to bring to a state of conscious awareness the outcomes of our actions and the beliefs and theories which are subsequently generated. The work of Schon (1987) and Polanyi (1962) supports Habermas' contention that the task of reflection is an integral part of human reasoning, but one which is often distorted by the very beliefs subjected to review. This issue has already been discussed in earlier reference to the difficulty families often have reconciling NDU practice with their expectations of the health service and care outcomes. In the NDU the task of critical reflection is to make sense of what happens in the NDU so that it can be increasingly anticipated.

NDU-focused research suggests that there are at least three forms or levels of communicative competence in use in the NDU.

- At the most basic level, communication is frustrated by the inability of an individual to verbalize, usually as a result of their physiological state but also as a result of advancing dementia. In these circumstances, understanding is reduced to the interpretation placed on the person's state as it presents through the other senses and as interpreted through the experience of the carer.
- Next, communicative competence may be influenced by a person's expectations of the NDU and what it has to offer. Frequently people at this level of communicative competence are referred to as 'ideal' residents, 'nice' family, 'good' nurses. They rarely challenge the status quo and are regularly observed to excuse omissions in practice, praising the commitment of staff and the wonderful service that is provided. Problems emerge for these people when the way they communicate does not reflect their real needs: either because of assumptions made about them by listeners – 'She/he doesn't really mean that. It's never a problem to him/her' – or because habits of mediocre communicative competence render the person unable to express their real feelings.
- The form of communicative competence most challenging to NDU members involves the communication of ideas and issues that challenge and confront the status quo. These communications include angry, frustrated outbursts and reasoned reflective critique of practice. In either case the effect is to hold up for scrutiny the

focus of such a communication and in this way either the issue or the way it has been interpreted or misrepresented becomes a focus for action.

Nursing interventions

The JFC NDU, in identifying its responsibility for developing nursing interventions, draws on Lydia Hall's concepts of care, core and cure as three processes that act to effect desired outcomes (Hall 1964). In terms of the BNDU model, the care, core and cure NDU interventions are considered as follows:

Care

Care is a concept essential to any health orientated definition of humanity. It is not a sole prerogative of nursing and individuals entering relationships founded on the development of mutuality in caring must be or become communicatively competent in order to best identify the respective contributions each has to make.

Core

Central to nursing practice, at its core, are nursing contributions to the activities of living commonly performed or controlled independently by people who have developed a need for nursing interventions. Johns (1991) identifies the potential reductionism inherent in using an activities of living framework for assessment and, at JFC, the BNDU model has been adapted to limit the potential for nursing assessment to reduce the assessed person to a series of actual and potential nursing tasks. At the same time, the Centre's Nursing Information System with its unique factorial design (Spry & O'Brien 1993) is based on activities of living and provides invaluable clinical and managerial data bases for developing, resourcing and monitoring nursing practice.

JFC NDU nurses are currently experimenting with an assessment format that is based on the cue questions suggested by Johns (1991). The intent is to develop a mechanism for interpretation of answers to questions that are person orientated, into activities that can be qualified in terms of their reasonableness as responses to the identified healing needs of individuals.

Cure

Curing is an intervention that can best be understood in its relationship to the process of triage. Whilst acknowledging that there are validity issues associated with Maslow's hierarchy of needs, the fact that the hierarchy is widely recognized amongst nurses has led to its being used as a framework for assessing the level at which interventions should be focused or prioritized from interaction to interaction. In the sense of paraphrasing Nightingale (1859, p.6), nursing should signify the proper use of resources, at the least expense of vital power to the patient. Curing in the NDU can be likened to the process of 'tuning in' to people's presenting needs and responding to their priorities rather than those of the nurse, to effect an early resolution of each presenting need.

Activities of living

The activities of living model used by the NDU (adopted from Henderson 1966), functions to identify necessary interventions and who should be involved whilst endeavouring through activities such as 'working and playing' to ensure that a sense of the person whose focus is the group's *raison d'être* is not subsumed by attention to a series of reductionist tasks.

The following summaries of three activities of living, as applied in the NDU, illustrate how the activities of living approach has been constructed in order to limit the potential reduction of each person to a series of task foci, whilst still providing an assessment framework from which to develop care plans. The intent is to provide foci for changing care strategies without losing sight of the person whose human needs are thus defined.

Activity: level of consciousness
    Considerations:
        Degree of awareness/alertness
        Post traumatic amnesia

- Glasgow coma scale ⎫
- Ranchos Los Amigos ⎬ levels of awareness

        Assume the resident can hear and understand the spoken word
        Note response to commands
        Note response to sound
        Call by preferred name
        Cognition levels – speech and occupational therapy reviews
        Stimulation – games and activities – occupational therapy assessment.

Activity: working/playing
    Considerations:

Provide home-like environment
Encourage normalization
Stimulation
Re-education
Family/significant other(s) involvement
Craft – recreation department
Home visits – occupational therapy assessment for wheelchair access
Rehabilitation is hard work
Outings and social visits/events
Recreation department – Centre bus for home visits and on-and
   off-campus activities
Relaxation classes
Attend multi-disciplinary team meetings regarding progress and future
   plan of care.

Activity: participation of family/significant other(s)
   Considerations:
      Part of the complete family unit – holistic care
      Part of the team – lay carers
      Support for the supporters – social worker, chaplain
      Regular access to meeting forums
      Education:

      ● tracheostomy care and management
      ● passive range of movement exercises
      ● 'brushing and icing exercises'
      ● gastrostomy feeding

      Attend multi-disciplinary team meetings with loved one
      Accompany loved one to Out-Patient Department appointments
      Arrange home visits – access cab (special adapted taxi service)
         or Centre bus
      Outings in Centre grounds.

The full list of activities used by the NDU are contrasted with Henderson's (1966) list to show how the NDU has identified activities of living
that may not be a regular focus for attention in common social settings
(Fig. 9.4).

Outcomes

The establishment of reflective nursing practice is intended to be the
focal outcome of the structure and process of NDU care because of its
ability to facilitate the achievement of strategic outcomes.

The NDU's activities of living	Henderson's activities of living
Breathing	Breathing
Mobilizing	Flexing
Communicating	Communicating
Eating and drinking	Eating and drinking
Eliminating	Eliminating
Level of awareness	Avoiding danger and injury
Safe environment	Sleeping and resting
Maintaining body temperature and blood pressure	Maintaining body temperature
Personal cleansing, dressing and grooming	Selecting clothes and dressing
Working/Playing	Cleaning and grooming
Expressing sexuality, role/altered body image	Working
Spiritual needs	Playing
Involving family/significant other(s)	Satisfying curiosity
Pain control	Worshipping

Fig. 9.4 Activities of living used by the NDU in contrast with Henderson's activities of living.

Social utility

The philosophical paradigm that underpins NDU patterns of practice is one of personal empowerment under extraordinarily disempowering circumstances. The issues that arise during the process of personal empowerment are numerous and to say outright that the NDU existing patterns of practice have optimal social utility would be a misrepresentation of the extent to which the Unit's commitment to its espoused philosophy is reflected in the emancipatory activities of NDU carers and residents. However, there has been a considerable body of evidence collected which suggests that positive care outcomes in the NDU are in fact the result of the form of caring that has been emplaced.

Other outcomes: research and quality assurance

The NDU has demonstrated its commitment to improving practice and the generation of new nursing knowledge in a number of ways and in a number of forums. The following sample is an indication of that commitment:

- Papers and poster presentations on NDU work and outcomes have been given in local, national and international forums.
- The NDU is currently involved in an action research project looking

at structure process and outcomes of care in four differing ward settings of the Centre.

- Post-graduate students of nursing have been invited to work with NDU staff and their work is fed back to inform the practice setting.
- NDU research projects completed and in progress include clinical trials of the EXACTECH glucometer, establishment of massage as a complementary nursing therapy, development of standards and criteria for care of tracheostomy and ventilator-reliant individuals, development of nursing protocols for skin care and wound management as well as a number of quality assurance exercises which include determination of the outcomes of social outings for residents plus auditing of ward management standards, standards of observed nursing care and nursing documentation.

The scope and diversity of this research endeavour reflect the unique contributions and individual interests of separate members of the NDU. Collectively the knowledge generated is filtered through NDU reflective processes and has contributed to an ever-increasing ability to articulate and portray the NDU's changing pattern of practice.

References

Brand, M. (1984) *Intending and Acting*. M.I.T. Press, London.

Fay, B. (1975) *Social Theory and Political Practice*. Unwin Hyman, Sydney.

Feild, L. & Winslow, E.H. (1985) Moving to a Nursing Model. *American Journal of Nursing*, **85**(10), 1100–101.

Glass, C. (1989) *Report of the Future Directions Working Party*, 1 & 2. Julia Farr Centre, Adelaide.

Greenwood, J. (1984) Nursing Research: A position paper. *Journal of Advanced Nursing*, **9**(1), 77–82.

Habermas, J. (1987) *Knowledge and Human Interests*, (translated by J. Shapiro). Polity Press, Cambridge.

Hall, L.E. (1964) Nursing – What is it? *The Canadian Nurse*, **60**(2), 150–54.

Henderson, V.A. (1966) *The nature of nursing: A definition and its implications for practice, research and education*. Macmillan, New York.

Johns, C.C. (1991) The Burford Nursing Development Unit holistic model of nursing practice. *Journal of Advanced Nursing*, **16**, 1090–98.

Johns, C.C. (1993) Professional supervision. *Journal of Nursing Management*, **1**(1), 9–18.

Kitson, A.L. (1987) A comparative analysis of lay-caring and professional (nursing) caring relationships. *International Journal of Nursing Studies*, **24**(2), 155–65.

McLaughlin, A.M. & Carey, J.L. (1993) The adversarial alliance: developing therapeutic relationships between families and the team in brain injury rehabilitation. *Brain Injury,* **7**(1), 45–59.

Newell, R. (1993) Anxiety, accuracy and reflection: The limits of professional development. *Journal of Advanced Nursing,* **17**, 1326–33.

Nightingale, F. (1859) *Notes on Nursing.* Harrison & Sons, London, reprinted by J.B. Lippincott Company, Philadelphia.

O'Brien, B.B. (1992) *An exploration of reflection and praxis: implications for nursing.* Published proceedings of the conference 'Nursing Research: Scholarship for Practice', Deakin University, Geelong, Australia, 1–2 July.

Polanyi, M. (1962) *Personal Knowledge.* Routledge & Kegan Paul, London.

Pusey, M. (1987) *Jurgen Habermas.* Ellis Horwood Ltd., Chichester, Sussex and Tavistock Publishers, London.

Schon, D.A. (1983) *The Reflective Practitioner: how professionals think in action.* Basic Books Inc., Publishers, New York.

Schon, D.A. (1987) *Educating the Reflective Practitioner: Towards a New Design for Teaching and Learning in the Professions.* Jossey-Bass Publishers, San Francisco.

Spry, J.M. & O'Brien, B.B. (1993) *Farrway: An interactive, computerised nursing information system.* Concurrent session presentation to International Council of Nurses 20th Quadrennial Congress, Madrid, Spain, 20–25 June.

Wright, S. (1989) Defining the Nursing Development Unit. *Nursing Standard,* **4**(7), 29–31.

Editor's commentary

This contribution offers a very different perspective from other contributions within the book; Bart O'Brien and Judith Pope have used the BNDU model to help reframe the way they view nursing at Julia Farr Centre in contrast with a critique of its use in practice.

The importance of this chapter is in trying to make sense of practice from a theoretical perspective thus creating a framework that is both meaningful and practical in the context of the care setting. Whether they succeed remains to be seen. However, there are clear tensions within this account, most notably the attempt to justify and modify a functionalist/systems approach through an activities of living framework within a fundamentally holistic perspective offered by the BNDU model. Their search for a more comprehensive framework is evident with the attempted integration of Lydia Hall's concepts of care, core, and cure and Maslow's hierarchy of needs. This mix of Hall and Maslow is open to philosophical scrutiny in terms of compatibility.

Perhaps this tension is, in part, created by adopting a revisionist approach, or in other words moving from what they already have rather than taking a completely fresh look at the philosophy and how it influences practice. The difficulty is that practitioners have current perceptions which need to be enhanced. Hence, there may need to be some qualitative leap to move people beyond their current perceptions. At Burford this was achieved with the development of a collective philosophy and at Julia Farr Centre with a cogent philosophy for practice which creates the opportunity for the 'qualitative leap' to move beyond their current eclectic functionalism. I raise the doubt to ensure future debate.

The answer is probably pragmatic: 'Does it lead to outcomes that are acceptable?' Within a critical reflective approach, as espoused within this chapter, such evaluative questions presumably are natural to address and resolve. Yet, if the model is to offer clear directions for research and the development of nursing knowledge such issues become significant.

Bart O'Brien and Judith Pope draw on critical theory to define concepts within their conceptual framework, reflecting on the resulting model's intended empowerment and emancipatory focus to enable practitioners to fulfil their therapeutic potential.

Critical theory has its own language with the result that Bart and Judith talk about similar concepts within the BNDU model using different language. For example, the concept of communicative competence at different levels is equated on the first level with the ability to establish the conditions which enable practitioners to work with patients and lay carers. At the second and third levels it is equated with the ability to fulfil collegial roles and to establish the conditions under which collegial relations and reciprocity between staff and lay carers can become a reality. The language used to express concepts within the BNDU model is important considering it always needs to be interpreted for personal meaning. Similarly, the concept of lay and professional discourses can be interpreted as recognizing that lay carers have different perspectives of caring to practitioners, and therefore there is a need to establish effective patterns of working with lay carers to enable mutual understanding of roles and purpose.

The core value of reflection within this chapter is very evident. The Julia Farr model has built into it reflective and evaluative mechanisms to ensure it is a constant and dynamic empowering agency. Practitioners must always pay attention to who they are and confront the contradictions within themselves in the face of experience and desirable practice.

Chapter 10
The View From Inside

Christopher Johns

The contributions in this book are about human caring as the essence of nursing practice. It is this fundamental belief in nursing as human caring that has led practitioners to explore how this belief can be expressed as a living reality through the development of the BNDU model. It is worth reiterating that the model is explicitly one of reflective practice. The cue questions form a model of structured reflection that aims to tune the practitioner into who the patient is within the context of the unit's shared beliefs and values and also who the practitioner is as a person.

The model is just one manifestation of reflection within practice at Burford, and latterly at Oxford Community Hospital. The value of reflection is that it offers the practitioners a window to look inside themselves. In doing so, 'who they are' becomes visible and enables the practitioners to come to understand 'who they are' in the context of their practice. This metaphoric window also enables the practitioners to look outside themselves at the world in order to make sense of it in terms of 'who they are' and their shared beliefs and values. In this sense it is a process of enlightenment (Fay 1987).

However, reflection is always action-orientated towards changing practice to resolve the contradictions between desired practice and the way practitioners actually practise. But why can't practitioners who have realized their beliefs and values just go out and practise in compatible ways? Why is this so profoundly difficult?

The reality is that nursing is constrained by an aggregate of powerful factors that act to limit the practitioners' therapeutic potential. These barriers are embedded and embodied in the traditions and culture of nursing. Whilst they can be understood, they are not amenable to rational change (Fay 1987). Hence, being enlightened does not necessarily bring with it correspondingly appropriate actions. It becomes necessary to create the conditions of practice that will facilitate desired practice. The BNDU model is one such condition of practice that can be seen as a liberating structure towards achieving desired practice.

However, in itself and by itself this model is merely a structure that promises much. Whilst the active participation of practitioners in formulating the BNDU model makes it immediately relevant and useful, it can simply be taken 'off the shelf' as with other models of nursing, and applied in an instrumental way, irrespective of contrary advice. The widespread instrumental approach to models is immediately recognizable as a significant barrier to using the BNDU model in practice as espoused within this book.

Yet again, the answer to this potential predicament may lie within the model. Even if it was to be used in an instrumental way, for example as an assessment strategy, it would still explicitly encourage practitioners to think about what it is they are doing, simply because it asks profound questions. No doubt such attempts will result in the 'cue' questions being interpreted as a rigid framework with significant gaps in patient assessment narratives concerned with such cue questions as, 'How does this person make me feel?', rather like the boxes concerned with sexuality and death that remained empty and silent in the practitioners' previous use of the Roper, Logan and Tierney model.

Similarly, the idea of 'narratives' as a way of recording information in a meaningful and useful way that builds on nursing's traditional oral mode of thinking, feeling and communicating about practice (Street 1991), involves a radical shift away from conceptualizing nursing practice within a nursing process format, even though the nursing process is meaningless to many practitioners. In considering such cue questions as, 'How can I help this person?', and, 'How does this person view the future?', the issues of outcomes can be readily envisaged. The more mundane technical aspects of care can be dealt with in packaged protocols.

Bart O'Brien and Judith Pope's account in Chapter 9 illustrates many of the complex issues involved in attempting to construct a compatible and internally consistent model for practice. Clearly it is not a simple process. But equally clearly it needs to be a simple process if practitioners are going to be 'sold' the notion that practice should be defined within a set of 'valid' philosophical beliefs about caring and its environmental context.

Yet the model can be used 'off the shelf', as initially utilized by Susan Metcalf in her district nursing practice (Chapter 8) with an intuitive feel that the concepts of caring within the model were a reflection of her own. But immediately, she began to reflect on what her beliefs and values were and her actions with her patients.

This suggests that a philosophy for practice is not an essential prerequisite for using the model in practice, but the model itself becomes the stimulus for developing such a philosophy. The reflective nature of the model inevitably demands that practitioners consider and articulate their own philosophies. But perhaps this is only true for those practitioners who are both willing and able to be reflective. The likely reality (and fear) is that practitioners will use the model like any other model, or indeed reject the model, because in comparison to other prescriptive models it may appear to lack the background of a complex mix of behavioural and natural sciences.

Brendan McCormack, Carol McCaffrey and Susan Booker's account of considering and using the model in practice (Chapter 6) highlights their intuitive use of the model. This intuition is based on an affinity of the model's beliefs and values with their own and it enables these to become visible and available for everyday practice. Carol McCaffrey's reflections illustrate a 'making sense' of using the model whilst using it in practice. In other words, applying the model does not have to be a considerable intellectual effort. Hence, the deceptive simplicity of the BNDU model is possibly its greatest strength.

The reflective nature of the model suggests that practitioners who intend to use this model will need to consider how they and their colleagues can become reflective. This may also be deceptively simple! It will be helpful if practitioners using the model spend time with each other at handover or in teaching sessions, sharing with each other the narratives they have written of patient care and exploring how this has been interpreted into proposed outcomes and actions.

As we have shown, practitioners at Burford and Oxford Community Hospital have used guided reflection to develop their nursing actions to become increasingly skilled in achieving defined therapeutic work (Johns 1993a; 1993b; 1994; Johns & Butcher 1993). Through reflection on everyday experiences, the assumptions and values embedded within the model are constantly reinforced in practice.

The model's assumptions

This may be an opportune moment to reiterate the model's assumptions as a form of summary:

- It is grounded in a cogent philosophy for practice.
- Nursing practice is underpinned by the unifying concept of human caring.
- Inside every nurse is a humanist struggling to get out.

- All nursing actions take place within the context of the nurse–patient relationship.
- It is a responsive and reflexive form in context with the environment in which it is practised.
- Practitioners are active and reflective creators of their own practice.

There are many other assumptions within this book concerning the BNDU model. In this respect it is more accurate to label these six concepts as 'first order assumptions'. Other assumptions are efforts to make these six more explicit.

I have striven to make the model internally consistent or, in other words, without contradiction. Yet I wonder if any attempt to make sense of such a complex concept as nursing can ever be free of contradiction. Perhaps contradictions are a reflection of our uncertainty and as such are healthy and should be welcomed. Perhaps the management of contradiction is the most profound common denominator of the way people and nurses lead their lives. Hence, contradiction is itself part of life.

The BNDU model seeks to help practitioners in finding greater meaning in their practice by helping them to unlock and liberate the caring instinct, and towards increasingly satisfying and fulfilling experiences for themselves and for the people they work with.

Informed moral passion

In referring to reflection as 'a window within the self', I am reminded of Jean Watson's 'commons room' in developing caring knowledge for nursing science and her plea for 'informed moral passion' as the landscape in which this commons room is situated (Watson 1990).

Models for nursing practice can be likened to 'common rooms' in the way they set out concepts as a room sets out its furniture, and how the concepts relate together as in the way the furniture is arranged, and how the concepts relate to practice as in the position of the room in relation to the landscape it exists within. Jean Watson states that this landscape needs to be open and fluid to respond to the constantly changing and evolving world of human science.

The BNDU model is informed moral passion. It is informed through the reflected lived experiences of practitioners who use it. It is moral through its explicit attention to the lived experiences of both practitioners and patients, and through its striving towards ever more effective and satisfying experiences. It is passionate in its stated assumptions, in its explicit attention to feelings and in its pursuance of nursing as human caring.

Validity

In Chapter 6, Brendan McCormack, Carol McCaffrey and Susan Booker scrutinize the validity of the BNDU model using a framework for the evaluation of theory in nursing (Meleis 1991). The model holds up well. Equally, it could be 'tested' against other well known criteria to demonstrate the strength of its validity as a conceptual model of nursing, for example, the (almost) universally agreed concepts of:

- the person receiving nursing
- the environment within which the person exists
- the health–illness continuum within which the person falls at the time of nursing intervention
- nursing actions/interventions. (Flaskerud & Halloran 1980)

These concepts are claimed to present a meta-paradigm of nursing (Fawcett 1984). McFarlane (1986) notes that a conceptual model is pre-theoretical, i.e. one which is not developed from empirical research and established theories. In fact, much criticism of conceptual models for nursing has been aimed at their lack of testing in practice situations. This in itself reflects an 'objective' approach to nursing practice – that it should be grounded in empirical research in the sense that practice can be explained, and predicted, and hence controlled.

But this approach is not a reflection of nursing as advocated within the beliefs and values of practitioners at Burford and elsewhere, where nursing is seen as a response to human need within the contexts of the particular practice situation and the nurse–patient relationship. As such, practitioners need models of nursing that facilitate their response to act in the most appropriate, congruent and consistent ways. Through reflection, the practitioners constantly 'test' the validity of the cue questions and the model for their practice. Hence, the model is emphatically grounded in empirical research, an empirical research based primarily on reflective, personal and intuitive knowledge constructed through everyday reflected experiences.

Through an analysis and comparison of practitioners' lived experiences in using the model in practice, an embedded and reflexive theory of practice emerges. This knowledge becomes another source of knowledge for the practitioners to assimilate into their personal practice through reflection, as with any other source of 'objective' or instrumental knowledge.

Hence, it becomes inconsequential to test the BNDU model against 'objective' criteria because such rules are irrelevant to the validity of the model. The validity is always through reflection on the practitioners' experiences – a process offered through the accounts in this book of the model in use. This is not to say that the 'universally' claimed concepts within the meta-paradigm are not useful as a focus for reflection. Without doubt, these concepts are comprehensively addressed, both explicitly and implicitly, within the model's concepts.

Neither am I suggesting a relativist position, i.e. a position that rejects that there are universal concepts and that nursing can be ultimately defined. It is evident through an understanding of nursing history that nursing is always changing/evolving in response to events. The BNDU model dynamically reflects this position at the micro level of actual practice, enabling practitioners to recognize, understand and respond to the multiple influences and events that impinge upon practice and to move towards achieving effective defined care.

References

Fawcett, J. (1984) *Analysis and Evaluation of Conceptual Models of Nursing.* Fred Davis, Philadelphia.

Fay, B. (1987) *Critical Social Science.* Polity Press, Cambridge.

Flaskerud, J.H. & Halloran, E.J. (1980) Areas of agreement in nursing theory development. *Advances in Nursing Science,* **3**(1), 1–7.

Johns, C.C. (1993a) Professional supervision. *Journal of Nursing Management,* **1**(1), 9–18.

Johns, C.C. (1993b) On becoming effective in ethical work. *Journal of Clinical Nursing,* **2**, 307–12.

Johns, C.C. (1994) Guided reflection. In *Reflective Practice in Nursing,* (eds A. Palmer, S. Burns & C. Bulman). Blackwell Scientific Publications, Oxford.

Johns, C.C. & Butcher, K. (1993) Learning through reflection: a case study of respite care. *Journal of Clinical Nursing,* **2**, 89–93.

McFarlane, J. (1986) The Value of Models for Care. In *Models for Nursing,* (eds B. Kershaw & J. Salvage), pp.1–6. John Wiley, Chichester.

Meleis, A.I. (1991) *Theoretical Nursing: Development & Progress.* J.B. Lippincott Company, Philadelphia.

Street, A.F. (1991) *Inside Nursing: A critical ethnography of nursing.* State University of New York Press, New York.

Watson, J. (1990) Caring knowledge and informed moral passion. *Advances in Nursing Science,* **13**(1), 15–24.

Appendix
Recording and Communicating Nursing Actions: BNDU Model Forms

Burford Community Hospital and Nursing Development Unit

BURFORD NURSING
DEVELOPMENT UNIT

PATIENT ASSESSMENT FORM : Personal Data

Patient.. D.O.B..

Wishes to be called...

Single/Married/Widowed/Other

Address of usual residence...

....Telephone No.:...

Family/others at this residence...

Next of kin..

Address..

Tel. Numbers (H)... (W)..

Significant others...

Religious Beliefs...

	Subsequent admissions	
Allergies:	Dates	Reason
Past Medical History		

GP	Tel.	PRIMARY NURSE

BNDU Holistic Model – Assessment Strategy:

Core Question
What information do I need to be able to nurse this person?

Cue questions:

Who is this person?

What health event brings the person into hospital?

How is this person feeling?

How has this event affected their usual life-patterns and roles?

How does this person make me feel?

How can I help this person?

What is important for this person to make their stay in hospital comfortable?

What support does this person have in life?

How do they view the future for themselves and others?

Burford Community Hospital and Nursing Development Unit

BURFORD NURSING DEVELOPMENT UNIT

PATIENT ASSESSMENT FORM : Nursing History

Date	

PATIENT: PRIMARY NURSE:

DATE OF ADMISSION:

NURSING CARE PLAN

Page

Date	No.	Problem/Need	Goal	Nursing Action	Prescribing Nurse's Signature	Date Review	Date Resolved or Plan Altered

NAME:

PRIMARY NURSE:

Special Intervention Sheet

NAME   PRIMARY NURSE

PROGRESS/EVALUATION NOTES

Date	Time	Prob. No.	PROGRESS/EVALUATION	SIGNATURE

NAME   PRIMARY NURSE

Burford Community Hospital and Nursing Development Unit

BURFORD NURSING DEVELOPMENT UNIT

DISCHARGE PLANNING SHEET

Patient.. Primary Nurse..

Referred Agencies	Contact	Referred Agencies	Contact

Burford Community Hospital and Nursing Development Unit

STANDARD: Discharge is managed to maximise patient and carer ability to cope.

Appendix i – policy for key actions/tasks of primary nurses.

1 Primary nurse writes a summarised care plan where continuity of nursing is required.

2 Primary nurse ensures all other workers are cognisant with the preparations for discharge.

3 Primary nurse identifies key worker for continued care of person. This will normally be either home care organiser or district nurse.

4 The key worker should visit the patient at least 7 days prior to envisaged date for discharge and discuss future care arrangements with the primary nurse.

5 Primary nurse decides to instigate a home visit. When this is decided she is responsible for co-ordinating appropriate health care/social care workers to effectively achieve this.

6 Primary nurse informs patient of likely discharge date at earliest possible time, and confirms date as soon as possible.

7 Primary nurse confirms the general practitioner has discharged the patient from medical treatment necessitating hospital management.

8 Primary nurse informs patient/relatives of rights to NHS hospital travel costs (H11).

9 Primary nurse ensures both patient and carer accept the discharge arrangements.

This policy negotiated and agreed by primary nurses at Burford Community Hospital, following consultation with other health care workers involved in hospital and community care of patients and relatives.

Index